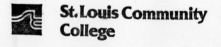

St. Louis Community College

Library

5801 Wilson Avenue
St. Louis, Missouri 63110

Straight Talk about Love and Sex for Teenagers

Straight Talk about Love and Sex for Teenagers

Jane Burgess-Kohn

Beacon Press   Boston

Copyright © 1979 by Jane Burgess-Kohn

Beacon Press books are published under the auspices of the Unitarian Universalist Association

Published simultaneously in Canada by Fitzhenry & Whiteside Limited, Toronto

All rights reserved

Printed in the United States of America

(hardcover) 9 8 7 6 5 4 3 2
(paperback) 9 8 7 6 5 4 3 2

Library of Congress Cataloging in Publication Data

Burgess-Kohn, Jane.
    Straight talk about love and sex for teenagers.

    Bibliography: p.
    Includes index.
    1. Sex instruction for youth. I. Title.
HQ35.B829   301.41′8′055   78-19603
ISBN 0-8070-2576-3
ISBN 0-8070-2577-1 pbk.

To my three-year-old granddaughter, Sarah Elizabeth Burgess,
with the hope that her generation will find sex education included
as a basic part of its school curriculum

acknowledgments

I WISH TO EXPRESS my deep appreciation to the high-school students who trusted me to provide answers to their questions and concerns. I would like to give my college students individual recognition for their willingness to share their emotions, experiences, and beliefs about love and sex. Because of the promise of anonymity and the large number of contributors, friends, and family members who gave me encouragement, I can only acknowledge my thanks and gratitude collectively to all those who made this book possible for me to write.

contents

introduction

THE FOCUS OF THIS BOOK is on you who are between the ages of sixteen and nineteen, and the decisions you make about your sexuality. I assume that you know most of the fundamentals about sex—basic anatomy, the changes your body has made through adolescence, the how of sexual intercourse, conception, and reproduction—and these topics are not discussed here in great detail. Instead, this book is more concerned with the thoughts, feelings, and questions that many of you have about love and sex. It is written to help you think through your feelings and make your own decisions about your sexuality—the decisions that are right for you as individuals, the decisions that *only you* can make.

For the past eleven years, I have been teaching marriage and family courses to college students, and lecturing to high-school students about dating, love, and sex. The material in this book is based on the questions that I have been asked by those high-school students and the discussions we have had, as well as the views and experiences of college students on sex-related topics.

From the questions I am asked, it seems to me that many of you are confused about dating, love, and sex. Certainly the way that sex is handled in our society perpetuates this confusion. On the one hand, sex is of prime interest to almost everyone. We talk about it constantly, buy titillating books about it, see it flaunted in magazines and on billboards, see it joked about on television, and joke about it ourselves. On the other hand, in our private lives, the subject of sex is often met with embarrassment, especially when brought up in serious conversation. The teenage daughter blushes; the father quickly changes the subject. As I'm sure many of you know, plain, open conversation about love and sex seldom occurs between parents and teenagers within most family circles. Yet I really think that if sex were talked about more openly, there wouldn't be so many misunderstandings in our society today.

Why is the subject of sex so difficult to discuss in most families? I am sure that many of your parents would like to tell you their views about love and sex, but they just can't break the barrier, the embarrassment that holds them back. Some parents actually are under the impression that you already know more than they about sex and are afraid you might show them up or become angry with them for thinking you don't know everything. Many parents, unfortunately, do not have the information about love and sex they need in order to inform you accurately.

Not only do parents find it difficult to talk with their children, but children in turn often feel awkward about asking personal questions of their parents. A close friend of mine who is a physician told me that when he tried to talk with his two young sons about the fundamentals of sex, they didn't want to discuss sex with him, and he had to ask one of his colleagues to talk to them. Very often boys and girls ask me personal questions that I know their parents would and could answer, but they tell me they feel uncomfortable talking about sex at home. Their own need for privacy often keeps them from talking with their parents about their sexual concerns.

Because of the way sex is handled in our society, it is easy to understand why many young people, as well as their parents, have come to believe that sex is dirty, that it is frightening or even dangerous. With such attitudes about sex, it is not surprising that parents and children have such difficulty discussing the subject. In order to instill and nourish in children a healthy attitude toward sex, parents *have* to learn how to communicate with their kids; children should be encouraged to go to them with their questions and get *straight* answers.

Very few of you teenagers today are getting the kinds of answers about love and sex that you really need. Perhaps you have had an experience similar to Susan's: "I wasn't told much at all by my parents. They must have expected me to find out elsewhere sooner or later, and I did. I think they would have talked more about it if I wanted them to, but I'm the one who was unwilling to discuss it with them. Now there doesn't seem to be any need to bring up the subject."

If you are a young woman, chances are that as you were approaching puberty you received some sex education about menstruation and reproduction—through a film at school in the fifth or sixth grade, through personal conversation, or through some books or pamphlets. Some of you may have been told about menstruation by your mothers, and probably reproduction was discussed, though perhaps without an explanation of the father's role in impregnating the egg. Most likely only a few of you received straight talk about sexual intercourse—the subject was left to your imagination!

If you are a boy, you probably have received even less information from your parents, and at a later age. Perhaps your parents gave you a book to read when you were in the seventh or eighth grade, a book that explained the changes that take place at puberty, such as how your voice changes and your pubic hair grows. A very fortunate few of you heard about a seminal emission—a wet dream—before its occurrence, or about masturbation as being a healthy activity. Or maybe your father offered you some pointers on how to act on a date—how to be a gentleman.

Boys often find it very difficult to engage their fathers in personal conversation. This is partly due to the fact that men have been conditioned to restrain their emotions in order to present a "macho" image. Seldom are men able to talk to each other at the intimate, emotional level that an honest discussion of sex requires.

Another reason why many fathers and sons cannot communicate readily about sex is that some fathers send out con-

flicting messages about their sons' sexual activities. While
they may very well expect and even encourage their sons to
go out and get sexual experience where they can, many
would rather guess the truth than know the fact, so they
refrain from any discussion of sexual intercourse or its consequences. Thus an awkward relationship can develop, in
which a son is confused about what his father expects of him.
At the same time, he is afraid to let his dad know his attitudes about sex. So Dad is not approached. Instead, older
brothers or sisters or friends are relied on for sexual information—and in many cases the accuracy of their information is
highly questionable.

But whether or not your parents actually have talked to
you in any detail about sex, you have developed some sexual
attitudes by perceiving their thoughts and feelings and actions about their own sexual relationships. If it is obvious to
you that your mother and father love each other, you probably have perceived love and sex as something that goes together beautifully with maturity. In addition, if you have
grown up in a warm, loving home where there is a feeling of
closeness, you are more likely to feel free to ask questions
and to receive honest answers. If, on the other hand, your
parents have behaved toward each other in an unfriendly
manner and have treated sex as something dirty, then you
may have developed a negative attitude toward the sexual
relationship between a man and a woman. In other words,
the relationship between your parents, as well as between
you and your parents, is crucial to the way you think about
sex.

If your parents cannot adequately give you the clinical
information you need, one might expect that the school
would be prepared to do the job. Occasionally an adult in
the school system will have the knowledge and ability to provide students with the kind of frank, honest, correct answers
they are looking for. Perhaps you have had a teacher such as
one past colleague of mine who told me, "I keep a file of
highly recommended books, written by reputable doctors
and sex educators on the topics of love, sex, contraceptives,

venereal disease, and marriage for my students to read. I
have been doing this for several years and no one has revealed
our little secret." Many adults argue for a sex education
program's being incorporated into the regular school curriculum and taught to all students along with math and English!
The chances are, however, that your school doesn't offer this.

It is clear that many of you have great difficulty in getting effective information about sex. For you who have not
found anyone to answer your questions, I am going to provide some straight answers. Feeling as I do, that those who
have been there can best tell it like it is, I have asked the advice of one hundred and twenty college freshmen and sopho-
mores in answering some of the questions that follow.

Straight Talk about Love and Sex for Teenagers

1 dating

DATING IS THE USUAL WAY to find a mate in our society. As you mature, you begin to notice the opposite sex, and dating becomes important to you. Suddenly you notice the boy next door in a different way. That girl whom you thought of as your *buddy* begins to attract you in other ways.

A date is primarily a recreational event in which two people spend a short period of time together. It does not involve any ties. A boy picks up a girl at her home at 7:30 on a Friday night, and their commitment ends when he returns her to her home at the end of the evening.

Dating is a means of learning about the opposite sex and how to behave with them. Interest develops between a boy and a girl through dating even though, at first, contacts may be clumsy and the two of you are often very unsure of how to behave toward each other. Sometimes early boy-girl relationships are made a little easier through group dating at such occasions as high-school parties and sports events. Going together in the *hit-or-miss* fashion teaches the importance and pleasure possible in dating. You discover the satisfaction of being *chosen* or *accepted* as a date. Success in dating also means success among your group of friends. It can also make you feel important to yourself. Dating is often the subject of conversation among friends and is a pleasurable part of growing up. It is full of freedom because it is done just for fun.

Most of you probably have parents who take an active interest in your dating, wanting to know your plans for the evening. Though your parents' interest comes from a general concern for your welfare and happiness, perhaps you find this interest meddlesome and old-fashioned. Your friends' ideas may seem far more important to you, and whom you date, where you go, what you wear, and what you do may be influenced more by what they say and do than what your parents would like.

Many young adults have complained to me that their parents seem to focus more on teenage sexual behavior and its consequences than on other aspects of dating. Many of you girls seem to hear what Anne, a student of mine, was told: "The only thing Mother ever said about dating was *behave.* I guess she thinks I'm going to do what she did when she was my age. She got pregnant.

"My father says nothing."

Virginia told me: "When I wanted to date, my mother coyly discussed the behavior of me and my date—don't go to *outdoor* movies, and come home right after the event. She never really warned or educated me about why I should and shouldn't do these things."

Jean's mother told her, "On the first couple of dates the boys will tell you anything, they'll sweet-talk you just to get down your pants. Don't let him, for a boy will like a girl more if she is decent—if she doesn't let him do anything." Jean wasn't told what might happen if the boy did get her pants down.

Young men more often receive advice about dating from their fathers. Tim told me, "At age fifteen, I was told how to go about dating. Dad said that if I liked a girl, I should call her up and ask her to go to a movie. He told me what to do and what not to do. I was not supposed to make a pass at my date the first time I took her out. If she seemed to expect a good-night kiss, that was okay. If she really seemed to like me and we turned on to each other, he said we should try petting for sexual release. I was also told by my father that sexual intercourse is great, but to make sure nobody gets hurt. She should want it, too, and I should not force her. I had sexual intercourse at fifteen with a casual friend. I'm glad my dad had taught me to use a condom."

Blake had a slightly different conversation with his

father: "At about seventeen, when I began seeing girls, quite often my father became very concerned about me becoming a father without first becoming a husband. No real specifics—generally just 'don't get into trouble,' without telling me how not to get in trouble."

It appears that most parents do worry about the sexual behavior of their children and the possible consequences. It is also clear that few parents are giving the necessary specifics about dating just for fun and not for sex. The following questions and answers provide some of this information. These questions have been asked by high-school students (mostly girls in this case); the answers include a sharing of the insights and experiences of college students.

What is the ideal age to start dating?

When to begin dating is an individual thing. The correct age varies with each person's attitudes and maturity. As a student of mine has written, "Each person matures at a different age and becomes interested in dating at a different time. You should start dating when you become interested in making serious friends with people of the opposite sex and feel that you are prepared to accept the burdens and responsibilities of more serious relationships with them."

Dating seems to be starting at younger and younger ages. There are some parents who encourage their very young children to date. Perhaps this gives a kind of boost to the parent's own self-importance. Others, knowing the immaturity of their children in handling emotional pressures, attempt to set limits on the age of that first date. This varies from family to family.

Students I have contacted indicate that most young people today begin dating somewhere between the ages of ten to fourteen. Many girls, however, have told me they are very sorry they had started "fooling around" with boys when they were just twelve or thirteen because they know now they were not mature enough to handle the pressures for more advanced sexual behavior from the boys they knew.

Some girls have told me they were surprised, too, at their inability to control their own sexual desires.

Jeanie, for example, told me, "I had always been taught that *good* girls don't get excited like boys do when they see pornography or watch sex acts in a movie. Since I knew I was a *good* girl, I had full confidence in myself to be able to flirt and tease a guy and still be a virgin. I was so wrong. One night after watching a very sexy movie with my date, I got so turned on that I wanted to make out with him. And I'm sorry to say, that night I was *easy* to persuade to have sexual intercourse. I still don't know what happened that I lost all sense of reason. I didn't even particularly like the guy!"

The fact is that our sexual desires as well as other emotional needs can be aroused in unpredictable ways and by unforeseen circumstances and factors. Research tells us that the age at which a child becomes sexually active is one of these factors.

Girls and boys who begin sexual activities at an early age are more likely to have intercourse before marriage. I discovered through my own study of high-school seniors and college freshmen that most of those who still have *not* had sexual intercourse waited until they were much older to have their first kiss with the opposite sex than did those students who *have* experienced sexual intercourse. For example, of the students who have had sexual intercourse, almost twice as many had their first kiss between the ages of five and fourteen, as compared with those who have abstained.

This same age differential was noted when I asked whether they had caressed another's breast or had had their breast caressed. Among the boys and girls who have experienced sexual intercourse, twice as many had also experienced light petting between the ages of ten and sixteen, in contrast with students who have not had sexual intercourse.

My study further showed that boys and girls who engage in *heavy petting* at an early age are likely to experience sexual intercourse at an early age. When asked if they had petted (caressed another's body in the genital areas), over

half the boys and girls who have *not* had sexual intercourse
had also not experienced heavy petting. On the other hand,
of those who *have* had intercourse, four times as many had
also experienced heavy petting by the age of fifteen, in
comparison to young people without the experience of
sexual intercourse. It is therefore clear that boys and girls
who engage in early sexual activity are more likely to progress to sexual intercourse.

For both sexes, it is, perhaps, best to wait until one is at
least fifteen or sixteen before dating. In our culture, boys
are usually older than girls when they begin dating because
of the practice of dating a girl younger than they. Also, since
it is customary for boys to pay for the expenses of a date,
they usually must be old enough to have some kind of job
before they can think of taking out girls.

But no matter what the "correct" age might be, no teenager should be pressured by friends or even anxious mothers
into too-early dating.

*How well should you know a guy before you accept a date
from him?*

It is not necessary to know a boy really well before accepting
a date from him. After all, one of the purposes of dating is to
have a chance to get to know someone better. As John has
said: "Your first date should be a chance to learn more about
the guy and form an opinion about further dates with him.
The important thing is to date. You're not going to get anywhere hiding in the corner and not meeting and knowing
other people. Of course, if you don't trust the guy at all, then
you shouldn't date him."

*When a guy asks you to go out for the first time, should you
ask what to wear?*

Most fellows I know answer no to this question. As Bill advised: "Wear what you want to wear. You should know what

kind of activity is planned, though. But use your common sense, because the way you dress on your first date tells him something about you."

I don't seem to be able to talk to guys when I go out with them. I was wondering what I could say that would be interesting.

Most young men seem to feel that girls on a date should try to find out what the fellow is interested in and talk to him about those things. But as Reg said: "You should also talk about yourself and things you are interested in so that the guy can get a better understanding of what you are like. Be natural—don't force yourself to talk about things you don't like or don't know anything about. If you relax and act like yourself, words will form."

Tim differed and said: "In our dating system, the boys usually feel that the conversation is up to them. If a boy is afraid and doesn't talk, a girl will not go out with him again. Leave the topics up to the guys, and let the conversations roll from there."

It is important to learn to communicate if you want to develop successful relationships with others. One of the things that make life worth living is the ability to respond to others in a warm, spontaneous manner, giving your friends the feeling that you care about their needs. I am sure that most people would like to respond in this way to those they like, but not everyone succeeds. Why? The answer is twofold:

Several factors determine human behavior—our intelligence potential; our temperament, which influences us to be slow or quick to anger and to forgive, to be outgoing or shy; our energy levels, which influence how active we will be and how much rest we need; and our many innate drives, such as the need for food, drink, and sex.

Second, the kind of family relationships we have and the way we have been reared are equally important influences on one's behavior. For example, if you were brought up in a home to feel embarrassed or awkward about your sexual feelings, you may feel the same way about dating. How can you be relaxed and *natural*, as Reg suggested, if you are hesitant or embarrassed about how to relate to a member of the opposite sex? If you are a very shy person and have never learned the art of conversation, how can you develop the necessary give and take that is an important part of the pleasant relationship? I don't agree with Tim, who suggested that girls should just let the boys decide the topics of conversation, or that girls won't go out again with boys who are afraid to talk.

In the first place, regardless of inborn potential or how one is reared in a family, everyone can learn to improve his or her own communication skills. And if you can make your date feel comfortable, even a shy boy or girl can be encouraged to converse. Personality changes are difficult to make, especially if one has always been bashful or unable to express thoughts and feelings, but they can be accomplished if one is determined.

First you must concentrate on your own behavior and know that when you are on a date you are completely responsible for what you do and say. If you want interesting conversation, be prepared before you go on a date. Find out things your date might be interested in talking about. Be confident in yourself. If he asked you for a date, he must have thought you attractive and fun to be with. If she accepted your invitation for a date, or asked you out, she thinks you are an okay guy!

Learn to share your thoughts and feelings with others. You want to be understood, and so does your partner. A relationship is reciprocal—a give-and-take affair. A person who is always talking about himself, or one who always has to have her own way without caring about how you feel, is not a very good companion to date. But, of course, in order for someone to understand you, you must make your likes and dislikes, your goals and values, very clear. If, for example, you have limited funds, don't ask your date where she would like to go and then become angry when she suggests a place far too expensive for you.

Communication, as I have said, is a give-and-take process in which you can learn to understand others and they can learn to understand you. The process of interchange involves the tone of our voice, gestures, smiles, frowns, other body movements, the way we dress. We make friends through nonverbal as well as verbal communication. If a girl wants to attract the attention of a boy, she can accomplish it through a pretty smile, pleasant facial expressions, showing she likes him, and a "Hello, wasn't that a good (or boring) discussion in class today?" Or, "After the game tonight I'm having some kids over, would you like to come, too?"

How do you become friends with guys if you are scared or shy and don't know how to establish a friendship? How do you catch a guy's eye?

Clearly, the best way to make friends with anybody is to act like yourself. As Will said: "Don't try to put on a front to impress him. Be yourself. If you pass him in the halls at school, say "Hi" and try to start a conversation. But don't be too pushy." Mike added: "Make yourself more available by going to parties and dances at school. By doing this, you will get over your fears and will meet new people who can lead into meaningful relationships."

Larry opted for a more straightforward approach: "If you like him, be completely frank and honest in letting him know your feelings. The best and probably easiest way to get a boy to ask you out is to come right out and ask him. If you're not that forward, however, become interested in what he's interested in, make yourself noticeable, but be careful not to become a showoff."

Why is so much more emphasis placed on physical attraction than on personality factors in dating?

Rick speaks for many young men: "It's hard to become attracted on the basis of personality when you have to get to know girls through dating to find out what they are like. Physical attraction is much easier to identify. But I do agree that too much emphasis is placed on a pretty face and figure."

The college girls I've queried say practically the same thing; they agree that physical attractiveness may be the spark that starts a relationship. But after that, they hope that personality would take precedence over a pretty face.

Our society places great emphasis on physical attractiveness. As Larry said, "Being seen with a really *cool chick* is a boost to a guy's ego." Of course, the important thing is that there be some kind of mutual attraction that causes two people to want to get better acquainted. One young man's fancy may turn to a pretty face; another's because of mutual interests in, let's say, sports or music. Physical attractiveness, personality factors, and social factors—all these tend to be reasons why people turn on to each other.

Should the boy make the first move toward a stable dating relationship?

Most of the college men agree that it is good for the girl to show she is interested, and then the boy will usually make the first move. As Tom said, "Some guys might *not* like the girl's making the first move, but I don't think most guys would really mind. A stable dating relationship involves two people, and therefore it is up to both partners to express themselves after they begin dating, not just the guy. I think it's really great for the girl to call the guy occasionally. This is one way for the girl to let the guy know he's not chasing down a dead-end street." It seems that most fellows do not object to girls calling them, especially after several dates.

Is it unusual for a girl to feel uncomfortable when a boy is near her and get nervous when he holds her hand or touches her? How far should a girl go with a guy when they are on their first date?

When a boy and a girl begin to date, they often lack self-confidence and certainly the know-how of dating, so they are very likely to be a bit unsure of themselves and, perhaps, a bit bashful. After a few dates, knowing what pleases makes going out easier and more pleasant. As Sue said, "At eighteen, I now have no trouble knowing what to do on a date. But when I first started dating at sixteen, I was really a mess—so unsure of what to wear and what to say. Then, I discovered that the guys were nervous on the first time too, and that made me feel better."

When you are sixteen, you may be more nervous or inhibited than you will be when you are nineteen; you may be a sexually aggressive person and like physical contact, or you may be a shy or timid person. Your values may be such that you believe that the first time you go out together you should go as far as you and your date want, or you may think that kissing and petting should be done only after you have known each other for a while.

Jean, a nineteen-year-old student, told me how she felt about her first date at sixteen, and how she feels now. "On that first date, I felt that a simple good-night kiss was enough. Many young kids of that age are nervous when having their first date, so the kiss is usually the first barrier to get over.

"Even if I didn't receive a good-night kiss, I didn't mind, however. The first date is still a period of adjusting to each other, and it is more important to feel comfortable with a person and not have to worry about the physical part. That should come later on in a relationship, no matter what peers are saying. I think that society talks about sex so much that it makes it even more uncomfortable to be around the opposite sex when you are sixteen. I guess my answer to the question of how far a girl should go would have to be a good-night kiss, because on the first date it is more important to talk and establish a comfortable situation than to see how far you can get.

"I think it really doesn't change once one is older. On my first dates, now that I am nineteen, I'm still nervous. It takes time for me to relax. I think if a guy would 'try' more than a kiss, it would turn me off, just because he doesn't show respect toward me.

"When people are nineteen, it doesn't mean they can

handle more than when they were sixteen. Once the first date is over and the second occurs, some nervousness is gone, but that still doesn't mean more should happen. For me, a relationship can't all be based on sex. I've watched my girlfriends have their problems and their abortions, just because they had the physical part and not the emotional part of a relationship. Seeing their agony makes me want a sound relationship not based entirely on sex.

"Sometimes I feel that my attitude about a relationship is really 'not with the times.' But then again, I feel that when I finally do establish a relationship, it will last longer just because I don't count on or rely fully on the physical part."

Most of the girls agreed that a good-night kiss is all right on that first date. The fellows agreed, too, although some felt that what happened was up to the couple. David at nineteen felt that it depends on your age and how you feel about each other. He said, "The first date I had with the girl I'm engaged to was terrific. I intended only to kiss her good-night and told her that I didn't usually do that on my first date. When our lips met, all hell broke loose—it was like magic and we felt an immediate sexual need for each other. I put my hands inside her blouse and caressed her breasts, and she fondled my penis. We stopped at that because neither of us believes in sexual intercourse before marriage. So all I can say is that it all depends on the couple."

Scott strongly disagrees. "I think a good-night kiss is fine on the first date, but beyond that, sex on the first date shows you that she is easy."

Should you act sexy on a date when you actually have no intention of letting him go very far?

Most male college students I've spoken with believe strongly that a girl should not lead a guy on if she has no intention of going further. As John said: "Being a tease is not going to help your relationship or your reputation. Flirting can turn a man on, and if you try to turn him off too late, you may be sorry about the outcome."

I have found that most girls, too, feel it very unfair for a girl to lead a boy on when she does not intend to get involved in a sexual relationship. As suggested earlier, often a girl has the notion that she can be strong and always keep the situation in control. This notion is a myth for young women in our present generation. The rise in the number of teenage pregnancies today gives a clear indication that girls today are often finding themselves as unable as boys to stop before sexual intercourse occurs. In 1970, there were approximately 400,000 births to unwed mothers; by 1980, predictions are for 500,000 illegitimate births. Premarital pregnancies are increasing fastest among girls under sixteen years of age! This indicates that girls cannot always hold the boy off once they become sexually aroused. (Or, of course, it may also mean that more girls don't want to resist.)

How can you tell guys that you only want to be friends and don't want to worry about cuddling or kissing? After all, sometimes you just want to go out for fun and not get serious.

As I mentioned earlier in this chapter, openness and honesty are essential to a healthy relationship. As Jim advises, "If you don't want to cuddle or kiss, just tell the guy. Just be direct and tell him. If he doesn't want to take you out anymore, look for other guys to go out with just to have fun. Explain your feelings; don't feel trapped and do something you'll regret later."

When sex is the main reason a boy takes out a girl, it will seldom lead to a relationship that can grow into something important and lasting. Sex, to be really beautiful, should be an expression of love and should reflect the respect, concern, and responsibility of two persons for each other.

Dating, as we have seen, is primarily fun. It requires no serious commitment. It may or may not include a casual sexual involvement.

As you grow older and nearer the age of selecting a mate,

dating will become more frequent and more important. It may turn into a situation of commitment when you want to share your life with someone on a more permanent basis. Then your thoughts will turn to love and going steady and, evolving from a noncommitted dating relationship, finding the "right" person will become an important concern.

2 falling in (and out of) love

WHEN YOU AND YOUR BOYFRIEND or girlfriend find
that you want to date each other exclusively, you may begin
to think seriously about going steady. Competing for dates
may suddenly lose its charm. You may find that you want
the sense of security you can get from having a commitment
with another person—knowing that you have someone to be
with, someone who wants to do things *only* with you. As
you continue a steady relationship, it may move from being
casual to becoming a fulfilling partnership. You may begin
to look at your partner as a potential mate and wonder if
this person is *really right* for you. Finding the "right" person is of crucial concern to most teenagers, and it is a primary reason why two people go steady.

What qualities make someone right?

Everyone seems to have his or her own ideas about what
makes someone *right.* But generally the right fellow or girl
is someone who is extremely compatible with you—someone
who shares *your* interests and basic values.
    So before you ask yourself if a particular person is right
for you, you should find out how well you know yourself.
What kind of person are you really? What sort of personality
do you have? What are your hopes for the future? What are
your interests? Your values? What do you need from another
person to make you happy? Can you empathize—see things
from your potential partner's point of view? Are you able
to make your partner feel good about herself or himself?
If you can answer such questions honestly, you may be
in a good position to figure out who can blend with you and
your personality to form a happy relationship.

14

The traits that make one couple right for each other may be very different from those that attract another couple. For instance, Jane, a young woman who works part-time in a neighborhood nursery school and is a tennis fanatic in her free time, says that a really right guy for her would be one who shares her interests in children and sports. "And he wouldn't be the jealous type, either," she said. "No, a right guy for me is not the jealous type because he has a good degree of emotional maturity—he is pretty grown-up."

Pam, on the other hand, has different priorities. She feels that a really right guy "thinks women are generally pretty nice. He respects women, and he is probably very nice to his mother and sisters. He is generally kind to others, especially those who are down and out. He is pretty easy to get along with, makes friends easily, and keeps them. He is known as an all-right guy. He considers his girl's feelings more than he does his own. He is not the kind of person who expects to get his own way all of the time, and he knows when his girlfriend is unhappy about giving in to him. When he gets angry, he does not just blame her for something without being willing to listen to reasons why it happened. He is understanding and forgiving."

And the right girl for Larry is "an optimistic person. She would be very kind to people and expect others to be kind, too. She would also be very cooperative and would want people around her to be happy. She would be understanding and slow to get angry. But when she was mad at you, you were sure to find out why and what for."

The traits most frequently mentioned among the college students I queried are: friendliness, honesty, trustworthiness, optimism, and a cheerful outlook on life. A happy person seems to make a happy mate. Similarity of interests and realism about life were also considered important by many.

How do you know if you have found the right *guy or girl?*

"You can really feel it if she is the right person for you," said Bill. "You feel comfortable with her, and your urge to look around is totally suppressed. The best way to know as much as possible about how you both feel about each other, however, is to be totally open and honest and to talk about the way you feel."

Jim added, "You can usually tell by the way you act with her whether or not she is right for you. If you enjoy being with her, smile a lot, and are generally happy, that's a good indication. If the two of you get irritable often and never or seldom want to do things together, you probably are not right for each other."

How long do you have to date someone before you know if you're made for each other?

Of course, there is no pat answer to this question. Finding out if you are "made for each other" is part of a process that depends on the development of a happy, healthy relationship between you and your partner. To know if you satisfy each other's need to feel secure and accepted, and to give each other a sense of belonging, a sense of well-being, takes time. The length of time depends to a great extent on how frank you can be with each other in discussing your differences and similarities—how you feel about sex, love, marriage, family.

The problems people have in really getting to know each other vary, according to the skills and understanding they have developed over the years. If you have had several dating experiences that have given you a chance to react to different kinds of personalities, if you have received good guidance in dealing with the peculiarities of others, and if you know your *own self* well, you will probably realize in a relatively short period of time whether or not you and your steady are really made for each other.

Most college men and women seem to feel that it would take at least a year for a couple to get to know each other *really* well, and several have said two or three years. But, as one student of mine has suggested, the important thing is to "give yourself enough time together before marriage to really get to know how both of you feel about finances, children, relatives, and sex, so that you can begin to work out differences even before marriage. This would give you a much better chance to make it work. If you have too many differences that you can't seem to work out during courtship, they will certainly cause trouble after marriage."

My girlfriend and I are going steady, but I don't want to always have to be with her. Why is it so hard for girls to accept the differences between us guys and themselves, such as differences in ideas about dating, going out with the guys, etc.?

Going steady does not mean *exclusive ownership*. In fact, too much togetherness can stifle a relationship; can stifle one's sense of individuality and cause one to feel trapped. We all find it pleasing to know we are loved and that someone likes to be with us. Knowing this should cause us to trust our partner enough to give him or her time and space to do things without us.

"A girl who thinks she wants a guy all to herself should remember that guys like to spend time with their friends, too," said Jake. "A girl sometimes feels that the guy doesn't like her if he misses taking her out just one night. She should accept the reality that we need some freedom to be with other friends and to do things on our own—even after marriage. It is wise to balance it out so that a guy and a girl will do many things together; yet each should do things with friends or family without the other along."

Anne expressed the view of many girls about a boyfriend's right to some free time to spend with his family and buddies. She said, "I know some girls who are very possessive of their boyfriends and react jealously if they don't have their complete attention."

As I suggested above, overpossessiveness of your future mate shows that there is an underlying lack of trust in your relationship. It indicates both immaturity and a lack of self-assurance—two very negative characteristics that you should bring under control, or they can cause many problems.

And this holds true as much for boys as for girls. A person who knows he or she is worthy of a partner's love and attention will not feel threatened or jealous when the partner is out of sight.

Why do I get jealous about my boyfriend? Isn't jealousy a sign of love? What can I do to get over feeling jealous?

It is only natural to experience some feelings of jealousy when you think you are being excluded from your partner's attention. When your partner pays attention to someone else, your first reaction often is to feel left out; you feel ignored, unappreciated. The thing to do when you feel jealous is to keep cool, and it will usually pass. But you might let him or her know you didn't like the attention given to someone else. For example, it would be all right to say, "I can't imagine what you and Pat could have found so interesting for such a long time," and then drop the subject.

It is another matter if you find that you or your partner remains upset or frequently reacts in a jealous or possessive way. As Jeri's experience shows, this kind of behavior can cause a relationship to dissolve: "I thought John really loved me when he behaved in his possessive, jealous manner. He would get mad at me for just smiling at another guy. But one time when he yelled and screamed at me right at a party, I said to him, 'What are you so afraid of?' He had such a low opinion of himself that he was constantly afraid I would leave him for someone else. After a while, it ceased to be fun to go with this guy. He was really neurotic. He had to maintain that *macho* image and demanded almost a slave attention from *his* girl.

"I began to realize that I didn't want to be stuck with a guy who had such little faith in himself that he couldn't trust me either. I *never* knew how he was going to behave and I got so I was afraid to say anything to him about how he made me feel with his constant accusations. I am a friendly person, and had no intention of ignoring all the rest of my friends to prove to this nerd that he was important to me.

He really wasn't a very happy person, and going out with him became a real drag.

"I feel sorry for him because his mom always favors his younger brother in every way, and so John just wants to be first with someone so bad that he overreacts. His brother is a football star; John can't make the team. His brother is real smart; John just seems to get by. And his family is always making comparisons. No wonder he is so susceptible to jealousy. No wonder he can be so cruel when he is not getting my undivided attention. But I don't owe him anything and I certainly wouldn't want to be married to such a man. He doesn't even want me to remain close to my family. So I told him I couldn't go with him anymore, and I am glad I did. I certainly am not smart enough to help him with his personality problems."

Jeri is quite correct in her assessment of John. Jealousy can be just a cry for more attention. But it can also be an indication of a deep-seated need for help to overcome feelings of insecurity and a low sense of self-esteem.

Demanding exclusive loyalty from another can be overcome if a person wants to work at it. If you are experiencing frequent bouts of jealousy, it would be wise for you to take a good look at yourself. How do you feel when you are jealous? What causes you to feel this way? How much control do you have over your own feelings?

If jealousy causes problems between you and your partner, you should have a long, open, honest talk with each other about your mutual needs, your limits, what you believe in. Talking is much better than remaining silent. It is less disruptive than shouting or violence. Be very specific about what you expect from the other person and what he or she can expect from you. It is certainly unrealistic ever to demand that your partner completely suppress affection for others.

If, after examining your feelings and discussing them with your partner, you discover that this jealousy and possessiveness is due to your insecurity or an inability to trust another to game playing or the desire to control your part-

ner, then it is time to recognize that a real problem exists.
It is time to think about making changes in your behavior
and your personality. This would take strong motivation
and perhaps psychiatric help. Whatever you decide about
your own jealousy or your partner's, it won't work unless
you *both* want to work at lessening these tendencies. You
won't succeed unless you *both* listen and talk to each other.
You need to be willing to confront the issue head-on. Jealousy is not a sign of love.

*I was so sure that I was in love with my girl when I first met
her, but I guess I didn't really know what love is. What is
love—the kind you should have when you want to settle
down?*

While many people still believe that something dramatic like
"love at first sight" can happen, they are usually mixing up
romantic attraction with love. There is a sharp difference
between the two: Romantic attraction can be instantaneous;
real love takes more time to develop.

Romance is an important aspect of going steady and finding love. Something happens to attract two people to each
other in the first place—a physical attractiveness (a pretty
or handsome face and figure) or a particular personality
shining through. I haven't found a definition for this *attraction* so I describe it as two persons being in tune with each
other like an instrumentalist and a vocalist blending into
each other's music to create a beautiful melody. This may be
an infatuation at first, but it may grow into love.

David gives a good example of a *real* love: "Donna is
beautiful and the first time I met her, I was very attracted
to her. I asked her for a date the very next day. In less than
a month, it was apparent to me that I loved her, but she was
much more slow in admitting her love for me. Our relationship progressed into a beautiful partnership and in six months
we were engaged. We knew it was love because we wanted the
commitment of marriage. We feel responsible for each other's

well-being and happiness, we share our thoughts, we respect
each other, we are happy together, but allow each other freedom to be with others and to do things alone, and we want
each other sexually. We are really in love."

As with other emotions, feelings of love vary for men and
women, and at different times in their relationship. Men are
said to fall *in* love faster than women, but once a woman has
decided she feels love for a man, she often is much more intense in showing him how much she loves him.

As stated earlier, when a man and a woman love each
other, they share feelings of care, respect, and responsibility
for the other. Their love includes sexual desire; it includes
a deep knowledge and understanding of each other. Love is
something we give as well as receive. If you know what love
is, then you can also learn *to* love, *to* care.

*What causes a relationship to go wrong? And how can you
gracefully end it?*

If you have any experience in dating you most likely have
experienced the ending of a relationship. This is often a very
difficult thing to deal with, especially for teenagers. The
longer the relationship has continued and the more intense
it has been, the more painful its ending may be.

Many romances are destined to end because of the reasons they began. You may not have chosen your dating partner wisely—you may have been too immature to form a
steady relationship. The attraction may have been primarily
sexual, especially if the girl gave off vibes that she was sexy,
or the boy only went into dating for sex. Usually the physical
attraction, which is falsely called love, will not sustain a relationship for long, if that is all there is.

Sally told me how she had ended a relationship that had
lasted several years: "We really believed that 'opposites attract' and at first our physical attraction was enough to keep
us together. Greg was the prize of the high-school campus—
prom king and all that. I was so proud to be his date. I didn't

want to be with anyone but him. He respected my wish not to have sexual intercourse, but we enjoyed real heavy petting a lot.

"After we had gone steady for a year, it seemed all we did was fight. We were so opposite in our likes and dislikes, and even in the way we felt about friends. We argued and quarreled about every little thing—which movie to see, what I was going to wear, whom he was talking to after class. I know I made impossible demands on his time trying to assure myself he really loved me.

"After we graduated from high school and I started college, he didn't seem so glamorous to me, clerking in a store. Many of the guys in college made me doubt my feelings about Greg. One day I accepted a date from a college classmate, and although I felt guilty, I realized that I no longer was satisfied or happy with Greg.

"My mother and sisters had always told me they thought I was wrong to go steady in high school. They also thought Greg was selfish and stuck on himself. I began to see they were not too wrong about him. But how do you end a relationship after going steady for two years!

"I decided to be frank with Greg. I told him that while I had truly enjoyed going steady, I knew we had lost interest in each other, and he agreed that our fighting all the time showed us we were too incompatible to get along. But he said he still loved and wanted me. I knew it would be difficult for him giving up the sexual part of our relationship, as it was for me. It was all very painful. Anyway, I insisted that we break up, at least for a while. Was I surprised to see how fast he was back in circulation again!

"After going with him for so long, I really didn't feel like getting involved right away again. Now, after three months, I am going on casual dates with guys I meet on the college campus. It was difficult to begin dating again after going steady, but I'm wiser and don't intend to get so emotionally involved so soon the next time. I want to be mature enough to be really ready for a good, lasting relationship after I graduate from college."

Ending a relationship is not the end of the world, even though it may seem so at the time. It will take time to get over it, but when you are a teenager, you have remarkable powers to recuperate. Each time you start a new relationship, you are learning more about yourself and the kind of person who will be right for you. People seldom perish from a broken heart over a broken engagement or going-steady affair.

Going steady is a commitment to exclude other members of the opposite sex as dates. It may mean the two people are in love, although for many younger teenagers love is not necessarily a factor. Couples may become sexually involved for various reasons. The next chapter discusses the decisions young people who date must make regarding premarital sex.

3 what about premarital sex?

IN MY OWN RESEARCH, which supports much of that
done by other sexologists and sociologists, I find that most
teenagers today believe that if two people are in love, it is
all right for them to engage in sexual intercourse outside marriage. Recent studies show that college students (approximately 83 percent) approve of premarital sex if the couple
is engaged or in love, and that about 40 percent of women
and 65 percent of men actually have experienced intercourse.[1] This is really not surprising, since girls and boys now
tend to mature earlier and marry later. Men and women are
beginning to feel and act sexually in similar ways. Girls have
more freedom today than ten years ago. Increasingly, they,
as well as boys, feel that premarital sex is all right in a stable,
affectionate dating relationship.

But what do you actually think is right for *you*? What do
you think about the value of waiting to have sexual intercourse until marriage? The following series of questions have
dominated the discussion sessions I have had with high-school
students through the years. The answers are not meant to
tell you what to do—to tell you what is right and what is
wrong—but instead to share with you experiences and insights from other young people who have recently faced
these questions themselves. In this way, you will find many
alternative answers to the questions or concerns you may
have about sexual behavior.

What exactly is premarital sex?

Premarital sex refers to sexual activities between a male and
female outside marriage. These activities are petting, including oral sex, and sexual intercourse.

Just what is petting?

When I ask college and high-school students to define petting for me, I am surprised by the variety of answers I receive:

"I would guess it means gently fondling your partner, but I suppose I have no idea really."

"To me, petting can be in degrees. Necking and caressing is the more reserved form, whereas anything up to oral sex is a heavier form."

"Sexual petting is caressing or fondling sex organs or other parts of the body. In the streets this is known as a *feel*."

"Petting, to me, means that both partners engage in touching each other's body. It can include any part of the body, but mainly it occurs on the breasts and around the vaginal area of a woman and around the chest and penis of a man. It does not matter whether the clothes are on or off."

"The early groping in the dark of the back seat of your old man's Dodge and the eager exploring hands of a young couple is what I always thought was petting. However, petting seems to be becoming a more affectionate word for foreplay. Heavy petting is usually very stimulating foreplay before sexual intercourse. But sticking your hands down some-body's pants doesn't mean that you will pull them off. Petting should not be confused with *feeling*, which is concerned mainly with the shoulders and breasts. Petting may be af-fectionate or exciting stroking of the back, thighs, head, face, neck, chest, breasts, and vaginal areas with the hands and the mouth. Petting is a very good way to give your girl an orgasm and to have one for yourself without having intercourse."

"I don't know. I guess it means touching. Maybe it's only holding hands."

"I read in a book once that petting is anything done below the waist, but I think it would include stroking the chest area of a girl. I really don't know; this is just what I think it is."

"Petting means the simple act of touching and explor-ing—not necessarily with someone emotionally close to you. It's not going all the way, but just satisfying your curiosity about different parts of the body of the person you are with.

Some feel that it usually leads to intercourse, but I feel this only happens if the person you are experimenting with is someone you are in love with."

"Petting can mean any kind of physical contact short of intercourse—touching, stroking, mutually masturbating, and other ways of pleasurable caressing, like kissing and fondling each other's penis and vaginal opening, which is called having oral sex."

"It brings you to orgasm. This leaves the girl breathless and happy and sexually satisfied without sexual intercourse. I don't know how it leaves the guy, but my boyfriend tells me that when I rub or suck his penis until he *comes* he is satisfied to wait for intercourse until we are married. Oral sex satisfies me, too."

Now that you have read the many definitions of petting, doesn't it seem wise when someone asks, "Do you go in for petting?" to find out what they mean? Clearly, *petting* means different things to different people. A good general definition of petting, however, is: all forms of physical contact with various parts of the body by using both the mouth and hands. It does not include sexual intercourse.

Does petting always lead to intercourse?

No, but it might. As Rob said, "Petting doesn't have to lead to anything if you don't want it to. You just have to stay within self-imposed limits. It is possible to pet for months without intercourse. My girlfriend and I masturbate each other and find we are very close to each other." Jim, on the other hand, said, "I'm more physical in bed, and so it is up to the girl to curb my activities. If she does not attempt to do so, then petting can lead to intercourse."

As petting gets more intense, it becomes more difficult for a couple to control their actions. "Petting is a wonderful way to show your love for each other," said Janet, "but you have to decide that this is far enough and then break off before you lose control. There are many ways to get sexual release and emotional satisfaction besides going into sexual intercourse. The mouth and hands can do marvelous things in bringing you to an orgasm."

"Petting," according to Nancy, "can be done for various reasons that do not necessarily lead to intercourse. It is true that sometimes petting is a kind of foreplay that builds up and climaxes in intercourse, but this is not always the case. Where an unwed couple is concerned, petting can release all of their sexual desires without the complications that sexual intercourse can bring about. I think petting is a good way to show your fondness for someone without fear of pregnancy, venereal disease, or loss of virginity."

Nancy is *not* quite correct. Petting can result in what is known as a *virgin birth*, though this is very rare. When a man rubs his penis against a woman's vulva without penetrating into her vagina, and he ejaculates, sperm can find its way up into her reproductive organs. The male sperm has a fast-acting tail and it can whip its way upward to meet an egg waiting in the woman's fallopian tube. This has happened even when the girl has her panties on!

Why do people think sex is dirty?

The idea grew out of our early-day religious and social sanctions toward sex as not being something one could and should enjoy. It was the Puritans of seventeenth-century New England who established our early sex values and regulations. Puritan love was a product of marriage, for love was the chief duty of husband and wife toward each other. Although being in love was not the primary reason for marriage, couples were advised not to wed unless they believed there was a strong possibility that a cordial love would develop.

Sexual union was considered the final step in marriage, and moderation was urged for both men and women. However, early Puritans were prone to forgive couples who could not restrain their sexual impulses until after marriage provided that their intent to marry had been announced in church. This announcement or "espousal" ceremony was

more binding than the modern engagement, and breaking
this commitment was considered adultery and punished as
such. Later on, the Roman Catholic Church had considerable
influence in the development of strict sanctions against premarital sex. Sex outside of marriage was declared sinful, and
most states declared this behavior illegal, even though theo-
retically there is separation of church and state.

In general, early religious attitudes about the sexual nature of women held that a *good* woman was to have sex only
in marriage. She would never admit to wanting or enjoying
sex. Men expressed their lusty sexual needs with *bad* women
outside of marriage. They had sex with their wives and probably enjoyed it, but intercourse was supposed to be done
only for reproduction. Sex was never to be talked about
openly by *nice* people. *So it must be dirty.* Generations have
passed down this embarrassed, furtive attitude about sex. For
example, in a book published in 1898, girls were told that
it was *self-abuse* to even imagine themselves enjoying the
embrace of a man before marriage! Such thoughts were considered evil habits.

Lack of proper sex education and society's habit of keeping talk of sex behind closed doors perpetuate these outdated
attitudes. As Liz, a student of mine, has said, "Society has
hid it from open discussion, causing it to become warped
and misleading. People think sex is dirty because they were
taught this by their parents, who were guilty, embarrassed,
and shameful about sex."

Today many parents still act as though sex is dirty for
their kids—if not for themselves. But changes have occurred,
and more resources are available for learning about sex as
a healthy, normal thing.

*Is is true that oral-genital sex is against the law in some
states?*

In 1974, the state of Illinois was the first to revise its sex
laws so that sexual gratification involving the sex organs of

one person and the mouth of another was no longer a criminal offense. Since then, few states have followed suit. Many sociologists and other concerned citizens, however, are still hoping that the rest of the country will revise sex laws to conform to present Illinois standards: protecting the individual from coercion; protecting children against sexual attacks by adults; prohibiting raw displays of sexual acts that would be upsetting to the public, but allowing acts committed between consenting adults.

Is there really anything wrong with oral-genital sex?

Whether oral sex is right or wrong depends upon one's own attitude and experience with it.

Not many of the college freshmen I have taught have experienced oral-genital contact. But Bob has, and he said: "Stimulating a girl by licking her genitals is terribly exciting and makes her have an orgasm very fast when we do get to intercourse. I used to think that doing this would be messy, but if the girl has bathed, her genitals taste as sweet as her mouth. I like my girl to suck on my penis, too, and I am always just as careful to clean my penis so that there is no chance of any secretions or smell to make it unpleasant for my girl *to go down on me.*"

Clearly, cleanliness is the key to enjoying oral sex. You wouldn't enjoy kissing a person who had bad breath; neither would you enjoy oral sex with an unclean, smelly sex organ.

Several girls in my classes who have experienced oral-genital sex tended to agree with an observation of Sally's: "I think genital kissing is wonderful, and it feels very exciting and really turns me on. It satisfies me, so that I don't need to have sexual intercourse. We call having an orgasm this way 'heavy petting.'"

Marie, on the other hand, thought the whole idea of oral-genital sex obnoxious and said: "I don't know how anyone can do this thing—it makes me sick to think about it."

What do you do if the guy wants you to go down on him (engage in oral-genital sex) and you don't want to?

Oral sex is an intimate act, as well as one that has been considered *unnatural* and *sinful* for anyone, including married persons. Thus, girls as well as boys may have strong feelings against it. Fondling your partner's penis with your mouth or having him kiss and mouth your vaginal area is an experience that must be willingly gone into.

Jean expressed the views of many teenage girls: "You tell the guy you aren't ready for this. If, after discussing your feelings with him, he still doesn't back off, you should find a boy who has more respect for your feelings and needs. Don't give in and try something that could really repel you if you are not emotionally ready for the act of oral sex."

All the young men considering this question agreed: "You talk it over with her, but as in sexual intercourse, you never try to force a girl into any sexual act."

What do you do when you want to have intercourse and your girlfriend does not?

If your girlfriend does not want to have sexual intercourse, she has her reasons—her morals, her desire to remain a virgin until marriage, her fear of pregnancy, whatever—and these reasons should be respected. Most college men and women I queried agree on this: Don't force the issue. "Find another outlet for sexual gratification," suggests Sam. "Masturbate. Or try petting. Whatever you do, don't force her into anything—respect her wishes. Have a long talk with her. Be respectful and loving and have patience. Maybe in time she will want to have sex as much as you. If she wants to wait until marriage, you may be a real lucky guy."

"Respect her wishes. Never rush into a sexual relationship," Karen emphasized. "If you love her, wait until she is ready. Unless you both agree, don't do it."

How far should you let a guy go when you have been going steady with him for a while?

This, of course, depends on your maturity—how well you are able to make a serious decision regarding your moral values and to accept the consequences of what you decide to do. Are you willing to risk the possible disrespect of your boyfriend if you agree to have intercourse? Can you handle the possibility of your own personal guilt?

Most college males I queried think that the answer depends on the individual and the situation. Whatever both feel comfortable in doing will depend upon each one's morals. As Dick said, "I feel it is not a matter of how far you let him go, but rather how much you stick by your own morals and how much he respects them."

Liz responded: "It's hard to say how far you should let him go. I think it depends upon your feelings toward the guy. If you feel comfortable with him and feel emotionally tied up with him, you'll know how far you'll want to go with him. It is a two-way street. If you lead him on, he will probably let you determine what is going to happen."

"If you have been going steady and are really in love," Jim adds, "you can improve your relationship with a sexual relationship. It ensures more love, trust, and respect in one another. Certainly there is no harm in sexual intercourse if you are going steady and planning to marry. Until then, know your limits."

Tom expressed a different opinion: "Refraining from sexual intercourse takes more courage and strength than giving in to your desires. Restraint expresses true love. When I was thirteen or fourteen, my mother gave me a book to read about sex. It told me I was doing the right thing by masturbating to take care of that ever-present erection I woke up with in the morning. All those stories about what can happen when you rub your penis to jack off were false. You don't get pimples, and it doesn't make you sterile so you can't father a child. I can resist sexual inter-

course by masturbating myself when I get home from a
date. Lately, my girl and I have been masturbating each
other."

*What do guys say about girls giving in to them on the first
date?*

David's comment is quite representative of the feelings most
young men seem to have on the subject: "She becomes
marked as an easy piece, and if I were the guy, I wouldn't
consider any lengthy relationship with her. Guys are likely
to brag openly about any girl they make on the first date,
which leads to a bad reputation for the girl. Fellows are very
likely to exaggerate, too, about easy girls."

Mark added: "I don't think a guy should *test* a girl's
morals, find them weak, and then look down upon her; he
is no better than she is for he tried to see how far he could
get. It seems nowadays to be an ego trip socially for a guy
to see how far he can go sexually with a girl."

"The girl becomes an instant sex object," said Al. "She
will probably get a lot of offers for dates, but nobody will
take her out with the intention of having a lasting relationship. Most will just date her for an easy score."

Jeri expresses the feelings of most girls: "Guys just make
fun of girls who go all the way on a first date. They run
your reputation down and label you loose and a one-night
stand, and then they don't want to be seen with you. Most
guys do tease each other about what they get and how they
got it. It boosts their ego."

Do boys always tell other guys about what they get?

According to the college freshmen I interviewed, some boys
tell, especially the immature kind; others don't tell. Sam,
for example, said, "I have had a variety of sexual relations
and I never discuss my personal affairs. Some fellows like
to brag and take this way to prove their masculinity."

How old should you be before you have intercourse? If love and sex together are the most beautiful things in life, why wait until marriage? I mean, if you love someone when you're seventeen, why shouldn't you show your love?

When you are emotionally mature enough to handle sex without guilt feelings and old enough to accept responsibilities for your actions, you are old enough to have sex. Perhaps you are mature enough at seventeen to enter into a sexual relationship. Some boys and girls no doubt do find that sexual intercourse is great fun. On the other hand, many young girls have discovered that taking a chance of getting pregnant is not worth any fun or popularity they might have. Boys who get sexually involved with a girl at seventeen are running the same risk as girls—pregnancy, venereal disease, being emotionally hurt, and getting the idea that sex is self-indulgence. Early sexual experiences are often very disappointing for the boy as well as the girl, because at sixteen or seventeen you are not mature enough for a deep, loving relationship, which is what sexual intercourse should be.

Janis summed this issue up very well when she said, "To have sex one should be old enough to understand fully the psychological implications about intercourse and why you are having it. You should be old enough to get contraceptives and to use them responsibly. You should also be old enough to be responsible about the possibility of a baby, to be able to care for it, quit school if necessary, marry—or to take the responsibility of an abortion—old enough to decide what is the best for everyone involved and to think about the future and the effects all of it could have on your life. The chronological age varies from person to person according to their maturity, but I would say anyone below eighteen years of age is absolutely not old enough."

Tom told me about his first sexual experience when he was seventeen. "She was seventeen, too, and had never

done it either. I couldn't get my penis hard, and when
I did, it didn't stay that way. Finally I got it in, and she
cried because it hurt her. We were both embarrassed by
this experience; I know it wasn't any fun for either of us.
And the agony when she told me that for all this mess
she was going to have a baby! Luckily, her parents helped
her give it up for adoption. We both felt so guilty—I, because I had done this and didn't really love her, and she,
because she brought such shame and embarrassment to
her parents."

Many young men I've talked with question whether
they, at seventeen, were really mature enough to know
the real meaning of love. As Rick said, "When I was seventeen, my understanding of love was not as deep as it is
now at twenty, and I believe that most of my friends would
agree with this. Just because you love someone doesn't
mean you have to have sex. I don't think sex is necessarily
wrong if you have a clear conception of what love really
is. But if you want to have intercourse as an expression
of your love, just make sure that it is love and not just
your sex drive."

And Roy added: "I feel that the decision to *make love*
should be determined by the true reality of the love relationship itself. At seventeen, it is more important to focus on
showing love by doing many things to make the other happy,
and, in time, sexual intercourse can become the extension of
that love."

Ruth expressed the views of many college girls when she
said: "Seventeen is too young to commit yourself to
one individual—a strong physical attraction does not gen-
erate love. At seventeen, a girl may feel she is in love, but
can she be sure her partner is not just engaging in a con-
quest?"

"Yes, it is wrong to have sexual intercourse at age seventeen," added Jan. "Even though you may really love the person, you have no assurance that love will last. What happens
if you fall in love with several other men before getting mar-

ried? Is it right to have sex with anyone and everyone you have strong feelings for?"

Martha, on the other hand, doesn't think it is entirely wrong to have sex at seventeen when you love someone. "But," she said, "if you *really* love someone, you have to look at all angles of what's going to take place and what may happen. You don't want to cause hurt or embarrassment for the one you love if a pregnancy occurs. Granted, you are physically ready for intercourse at seventeen, but are you emotionally ready to handle the guilt or the consequences that often come with premarital intercourse? If you're not sure of this, but still want to have intercourse with the guy you love, then it's time to discuss birth control with him and your doctor *before* it's too late."

Amy was seventeen when she first experienced sexual intercourse, and from what she tells about it, it appears that seventeen often is too young. "I was really flattered by the attention given me by a guy who was a sophomore in college. I didn't see him often, but whenever he came home, we dated. We would spend the whole evening kissing, and he would fondle my breasts with his hands. I enjoyed all this because it meant that we liked each other. Sometimes he would whisper that he wanted all of me. But I never wanted anything more than the petting we were doing, so I would just ignore him when he said these things.

"Then, during the summer, he started going with another girl who had the reputation of giving a guy anything he wanted. I missed him so much! Then one Saturday night, he asked me for a date. We went dancing and on the way home, we parked in our favorite spot beside a little lake in the country. We began to kiss each other, and when he said that I should prove I loved him and he would keep on seeing me, I agreed to it. I didn't even love him, and I didn't need sex, but I let him put his penis into me. I didn't feel anything, except that it hurt bad—so bad that I bled. In just a few moments it was all over, and he said with some disgust, 'You didn't respond at all; you didn't even act as though you enjoyed it—so forget it.' When he noticed the blood on his handkerchief he said he was sorry that he had done this to me.

"The whole thing was nothing but a mess. And now I was no longer a virgin, and I was angry and scared about that. What if I really did fall in love with a man, and he asked me if I was still a virgin and didn't want me if I wasn't? I was so filled with guilt about what I had done, just on impulse and for no real need.

"On Sunday morning I didn't think I could face my parents. I was sure I must look *different* and that they would know. I couldn't go to church because I felt so bad and wicked. I told my parents I didn't feel well, and they were so damn nice to me I wanted to cry out and ask them to forgive me, but I didn't because I really didn't want them to know what I had done.

"I didn't get asked for another date from my college friend, and I didn't want one either. I just hoped he wouldn't talk about it to his friends. Maybe he wouldn't, since he was responsible enough to use a condom so I couldn't get pregnant; maybe he would keep our affair to himself."

In having premarital sex, how do you know if the guy really does love you or if you're being played for a sucker? I just don't understand how you can know for sure.

You might answer this question yourself. How long have you known each other? Love is something that develops slowly as you get to know someone. How often do you see each other? When you are really in love you find that you want to be together as much as possible and if you are not, you are writing letters or calling on the phone. Amy is a good example of a girl who was played for a sucker. As you read about her experience, it was, I'm sure, obvious to you that hers was not a loving relationship.

How do you know it's love and not exploitation? Let's turn to what some college students have to say.

"There is no way to tell if the guy really loves you or is using you to satisfy his sex drive," said Dick. "You will just have to play it by the emotions exchanged. I know many guys that will play a woman for a sucker, but I also know just as many who are sincere in their relationships. I say that she had better not have premarital sex unless she knows without a doubt that he loves her for real. If she can't see how she could know, then she should know that this is reason enough *not* to have sex. If the guy does love you, he will wait until you are ready. Develop a relationship—talk freely and have confidence in each other. If putting him off sexually several times causes him to quit dating you, you have your answer— he was playing you for sex, not love. If he continues to date you, he has respect for you, and eventually this will grow into love."

It takes time to develop the kind of understanding and trust that forms the basis for love. Love requires emotional maturity. As Karen said, "Your partner should show the kind of love that demonstrates that he respects you. Does he like being with you? Does he spend time with you, or only when he wants your body? All these concerns enter into the picture of love. If you know that much about him and yourself, then make the choice. It's yours to make. People can influence you, but the decision is yours if you are honest and mature enough to handle the situation."

What is the difference between love and sex?

While most of you seem to have a strong notion that love and sex ought to go together, you also seem somewhat unclear as to the difference between love and sex. We have already defined love as being productive. Or, as Eric Fromm says in *The Art of Loving*, to love means to labor for someone—to do something to make another happy. Love is defined by others as a never-ending emotion, while sex is a physical drive. Once the sex drive is satisfied through sexual release, it is gone until the next time the need for a sexual release is there; whereas the feeling of love we have for our partner becomes even more intense.

The sexual drive is a very powerful force that usually requires the response of another person for its release. When you have intercourse with the person you love then you truly have experienced a meaningful interpersonal relationship. But it is not love when a fellow says, "If you really love me, then go all the way and prove it." This is exploitation.

I find it interesting that most college students with whom I have discussed sex feel that a boy who *really* loves a girl will not take advantage of her—he will not be likely to push a girl into having sexual intercourse when she is still a teenager because of the many hurts that can come to her. They also feel that boys who think of nothing but sex and fun, rather than sex and love, are immature and will regret their adventures as they grow older.

Is it true that boys are more interested in sex than in love and that girls are more interested in love than in sex?

To understand why a young man may be more interested in sex than love it is necessary to comprehend the differences in the biological and psychological make-ups of the male and female. Certainly both males and females become sexually excited; the sex drive in girls is as strong as it is in boys. But, generally, young men become sexually excited more easily than do girls, and they may respond to different kinds of physical and psychological stimulation.

The male testicles produce sperm constantly, which is then stored in the seminal vesicles until ejaculation. When these glands become full, pressure is felt in the penis, and to relieve this pressure, there is often an automatic erection of the penis, and the semen (which is a mixture of sperm and other glandular fluids) is ejaculated, usually during sleep in what is called a nocturnal emission or a *wet dream*. This process is the same that occurs during sexual intercourse or masturbation. Sexual tension is relieved through ejaculation of the semen and sperm from the penis. When this physiological tension or pressure is high, it does not take much to arouse a male sexually—pretty legs, bra-less girls in tight sweaters or blouses, or flirtatious mannerisms. Thus, a girl who acts overly interested in a fellow may turn him on sexually rather easily, and once turned on, he may find his desires difficult to turn off.

This, then, illustrates a fundamental difference between young men and women—the more *immediate* physiological tension brought on by natural processes in the male's body. This is not to say that teenage girls are not sexually aroused at the physical level, but it is felt that at that age they are more likely to be aroused psychologically than from physiological tension. But the different attitudes boys and girls seem to have about sex and love are due to other factors besides physical ones—environmental factors. The way boys and girls are raised in our society encourages these attitudes.

From the moment of birth, little boys and girls are treated differently as far as their sexuality goes. Little girls are taught that femininity means to cry, to be affectionate, to be tender. As they grow older, they may pick up the notion that good little girls aren't interested in sex, and they are encouraged to control any sexual feelings they might have. Generally, boys are not taught to control their sex drive, and they are often not encouraged to be sensitive to the feelings of others. Frequently they aren't even allowed to cry when they are little because crying is thought to be unmanly. It is not surprising that anyone who is brought up thinking that tenderness is bad is likely to think of sex as separate from love—to view sex as some kind of game rather than as an interpersonal relationship.

When either a boy or a girl has grown up feeling unloved or inferior about himself, sex can become an ego boost. For example, Tim's dad made him feel bad about himself because he wasn't big enough to make the football team. So, to build up his ego, his sense of importance, Tim set out to conquer sexually any girl he could. At least, his father would give him credit for that!

Ellen was fat and unattractive as a high-school sophomore. Her big desire was to be wanted by a young man. When a boy in her class made advances to her, she readily involved herself sexually with him. No one gave her much credit for this behavior. Yet, Tim's dad acted quite proud of his son— scoring with the gals.

We call this the *double standard*, and a young man brought up under this standard (to think that being tender and loving is unmanly, to seek sex to boost his ego) may try to talk even a girl he likes quite well into having intercourse and then lose interest in her as a potential marriage partner because she didn't say no. Now he can't be quite sure about her, and that is a risk any girl takes when she says yes.

A boy runs a risk, too, when he pushes for sexual intercourse, at the same time expecting his partner to control both her emotions and his sex desire. A girl very much in need of love, affection, attention from someone, a girl very much in love with a young man, a girl with a hostile feeling toward her parents and wanting to *show them*, or one with a strong physical sex drive—any one of these girls might find it very difficult to hold the line—to say no. Which is stronger? Emotional needs? Physical needs? I wouldn't want to say which. Both are potential arousal forces. Therefore, both sexes have problems in controlling their sexual behavior. Too often, I fear, young men misinterpret a girl's offer of affection as a desire for sex and will push her into intercourse.

Some high-school-age men, biologically at the peak of their sex drive, desire sex simply for release from physical tension. Some are interested in it just for the hell of it. Some, of course, are emotionally mature enough to want sex as an expression of love.

High-school-age girls may not get sexually aroused to the point that they must have physical release from sexual tension. It is my guess that most girls have a strong drive to do something—to give something of themselves to another person. Much of this is due to the way they are raised in our society, as we have seen. They may be looking for a feeling of being important to another person—and for this they will give sex. Some girls may attempt to win a person who appeals to them through sex. Like Amy, some may even try to rebuild a faltering relationship through sex. But no girl can be getting into a deep emotional relationship with a young man whose primary interest is physical sex. Usually, young people will find that sex without real love is not a very strong bond to hold a person.

In our society having premarital sex is considered wrong, but I don't feel this way, and neither does my boyfriend. We don't have intercourse, but we feel that this is one of the ways to express love for each other. Is there really any danger in doing this now; after all, we are planning on getting married.

No one can answer this for another person. Many couples who plan to get married do engage in sexual intercourse and find their relationship enhanced. Others find satisfaction in waiting until their wedding night. As one girl said, "Consummation of your marriage on your wedding night makes the wait worthwhile. It was beautiful, and having done heavy petting, we already had that feeling of intimacy. We had so looked forward to the moment when it was right for us to go all the way and we will never forget that moment on our wedding night."

A good, loving, trusting premarital sexual relationship, with or without sexual intercourse, can help a marriage. Sexual intercourse affected by guilt or a bad experience can hurt a marriage. There is no simple answer to this.

Most young men I've talked with feel that there is no real danger, provided certain stipulations are met. John, for example, said: "For me, I believe that premarital sex is a very

natural, big step toward the intimacy required for a successful marriage. A person can find out very much about another
in bed that would never be revealed on a less intimate level.
This revelation is not merely of the body but of the mind.
After intercourse and during afterplay, I find it much easier
to talk of hopes and dreams, fantasies and emotions that just
can't be explained or revealed with as good an understanding
before intercourse."

Will added, "But *premarital sex is wrong* if both parties
don't willingly consent, if both parties don't have first a
mutual affection, attraction, and respect for each other, and
if both parties don't agree on contraceptive measures to ensure that neither is hurt by an unwanted pregnancy. Fellows
can suffer deep emotional harm, too, if a girl rejects him after
being so close. I went to pieces after my girl threw me over. I
loved her, and thought she loved me."

Young women seem not to be so sure about the positive
aspects of premarital sex. Many of them reflect June's point
of view: "I think premarital sex can do extreme harm to any
person who engages in it. It doesn't necessarily have to do
harm, but I believe it can. If, after having sex, the girl becomes pregnant or the boy decides he no longer is interested
in the girl, serious emotional problems can arise. Premarital sex
gives no guarantees; therefore, many dreams can be shattered
because people's expectations are not fulfilled."

Susan expressed another view toward premarital sex: "In
order for two people to engage in premarital sex, I think they
should be sure of their love. The girl has to be sure that the
boy is not using her. The attraction should not be purely
physical, but deeply emotional. I think that if you are engaged, each one has made a commitment to the other that
should last throughout the years. It is my feeling that a sincere and loving bond between two people would be enhanced
by sharing love through sexual experiences.

"On the other hand, without love and proper birth control," she warned, "VD can be a possible danger and there is
always the danger of pregnancy. You should always be prepared to take responsibility for your actions."

But doesn't premarital sex actually help prepare you for marriage?

If sex was all there is to marriage, I might be inclined to say yes to this question. But even sex changes somewhat with marriage, when you can relax more completely, knowing that everyone approves, that you don't have to worry about being caught, that a pregnancy, although maybe not planned, would not be quite as devastating. After marriage, you are more likely to be sure of each other and thus to feel more free to tell your partner what you like or don't like about sex, and this will enhance the sexual relationship, even if it already is very satisfactory.

Marriage, as most of you realize, is much more than a sexual relationship. Research on this question shows that premarital sex does not significantly influence the chances for a lasting, happy marriage. When married couples have been studied, almost the same number of couples who had premarital sexual intercourse claimed a happy or unhappy marriage as those who waited for intercourse until they were wed.

"Premarital sex might give you sexual experience, but I see no preparation for marriage in it," warned John. Marriage involves earning a living, paying bills, being a good companion to a wife, caring for children. The greatest sex jock can still make a lousy husband."

Said Kathy, "Marriage, as a rule, means the elimination of guilt from sex and the freedom to have meaningful sex relations. Premarital sex can prepare you for marriage, depending on whether or not you think premarital experience has contributed to the quality of your lovemaking. But it's not necessary for a good marriage. If premarital sex were looked upon as all right by society, where would our country's morals be? Then, you may as well have sex when you're ten or twelve. Love and sex is a mature subject and should be dealt with as such when you're ready for it. It should not take place just because you are engaged or because it is the thing to do. It may not be right for you if you jump into it without lots of serious thought."

She continued: "There are other ways of showing love besides sexual intercourse. Much more meaningful ways, such as caring and sharing. Kissing and petting can also be a complete act of love if you want it to be felt that way."

Another student of mine, Marge, doesn't believe premarital sex prepares one for marriage. She says: "I think premarital sex can prepare you for *sex* in marriage, but not for marriage itself. Although sex is a very important part of marriage, marriage is more than sex. Marriage comes with a lot of responsibilities, and premarital sex doesn't prepare you for those responsibilities."

Rita added that her experience with premarital sex was great fun. "However, there was always the hurrying up, the fear of getting caught, of getting pregnant. Now that I'm married, with my guilt and fears gone, I can say our sex life bears little resemblance to premarital sex. It was frustrating not having an orgasm—now we have time to play around until I do!"

If you have had sexual intercourse with a guy and he begins to lose interest in you, what should you do?

Unfortunately, there isn't much that a girl can do when a boy loses interest in her, but to realize she made a mistake and to think harder before going into another relationship. There are many reasons, as we discussed earlier, for falling in and out of a dating relationship. Some boys find having intercourse a mess they didn't bargain for and want to break off with the girl. Some guys are exploiters and like to go from girl to girl without any serious commitment. As Janis said, "Try to talk out the situation and if this doesn't work, dump him—chalk one up for experience. Move on, but know the next guy much better before falling into this kind of empty relationship again."

Can premarital sex harm a girl socially?

Unfortunately, yes, due to the old double standard. When boys start to consider a certain girl to be easy, the rumors can spread very fast. If the girl gets a bad reputation, it can harm her for a long time. She will find that boys will want to use her for sex only, and will not be interested in building a long-lasting relationship. Of course this tends to happen more in the case of a girl who is promiscuous. The reaction is not so strong in the case of girls who have engaged in sexual intercourse with boys they have gone steady with for a long time.

I've gone out with lots of guys, but they're all the same. If I tell them to take their hands off me, it really turns them off. Is there any way you can turn down a guy's wanting something, without that guy thinking you are square?

This question brought out a variety of responses from young men. Mac gave a three-part answer: "First, decide what your values are concerning sex. Second, when a boy attempts to involve you in premarital sex, voice your objections in an honest and understanding way, attempt to make him see your personal feelings when you refuse. Third, if this does not work, then the boy has no respect for you as a person or friend, so drop him and stick to your convictions."

Gary became very angry at the implications to this question. He said, *"All guys are not the same.* Only a very insecure gal would even think she has to give in to pressure. If you have a good reputation, I think you can have enjoyable relationships without going all the way. If a girl tells a fellow she does not believe in premarital sex and does not flirt and tease as though she is interested in more, the boy will almost welcome or expect the rejection of further sexual endeavor."

Tom concluded: "It's quite obvious that a guy trying to get as much as he can is just using a gal. If he has any feeling or respect for his girl, he will gladly stop what he's trying to do and apologize for being a real *horn.*"

"Try to find somebody that can give you good information about sex," suggests Chuck. "Maybe you could give in a little to petting and find out what it's like, but if he keeps pressuring you, tell him to get lost because he does not love you for yourself, but only for your body. Just make sure you let him know you are interested in him, but have no interest in sex at this time."

"I think it's great that some girls have the guts and maturity to wait for sex with the right guy," said another young man. "A girl shouldn't even want to go out with a guy if all he wants is sex. A guy worth getting serious about will be one that sees more in a girl than mere sex. Because you tell a guy you will go on a date with him does not mean you have to go to bed with him!"

Most girls replied that girls should *not* be afraid to stand up for what they believe. As Sarah said, "Be honest with your feelings. If he is worth anything, he'll understand and respect you. But don't turn him down completely—settle for a happy medium such as petting without intercourse. And remember that a girl must not tease a guy if she does not intend to give."

Julie represents the views of many girls as she tells us: "A lot of guys respect a girl because she wants to wait until marriage. Many men would feel proud to be that first man, but most men don't admit it; they want to be men *now*. They don't want to be turned down, and, in turn, their ego gets hurt and they react accordingly—as if you're not normal for refusing.

"All you can do when you turn him down is sweetly and maturely explain your feelings about premarital sexual intercourse. Tell him you're flattered by the invitation, but you don't feel ready. If he still acts hostile or doesn't understand, he's not worth going out with. Or maybe you have been hanging around the wrong guys. Just wait until you find a man who is willing to wait until he marries you to have sex."

I'm a guy who believes in the old-fashioned idea of courtship—that is, marriage before sex. None of the other guys I know think that way, and they make fun of me. Is this desire to wait really so strange?

Everyone doesn't have the same idea; some men do feel strongly about waiting until marriage to have sexual intercourse. As Rick said: "Stick to your guns about not having sex. My girlfriend is a virgin, and we've been going together for over six months. I love and respect her, and she loves and respects me. I will marry her, for she has the qualities I've always wanted in a wife. If there is not love and respect and unselfishness in the relationship, don't count on it to last. Sex does not buy love, nor does love buy sex. Sex is an expression of love and respect and is most beautiful in marriage."

Most girls I queried feel they would respect a guy who would be willing to wait for sex until marriage. They, too, said if a boy believes in abstinence, he should stick to his beliefs. As Nancy said, "Eventually you'll find a girl worthy of your love and not like the girls who are easy to make."

Where can a teenage couple go for help when they have been having sex relations for one-and-a-half years and the girl hasn't had an orgasm? What is an orgasm exactly? Is it necessary in order to enjoy sex?

Sexologists have thought that the most significant block to having an orgasm for a woman is psychological. When she feels embarrassed or guilty, a woman cannot abandon herself to having sexual release. Fear of pregnancy can also inhibit a woman's giving herself to the pleasure of the sex act so that she can reach orgasm.

An orgasm is a highly pleasurable, seizure-like response that generally lasts about four to ten seconds. (Some describe it as a big sneeze in the vagina.) The sensation happens in the center of the pelvic area—the clitoris and vulva for a woman (and the penis and prostate for men).

The _key_ to a woman's orgasm is the clitoris. It is a myth that orgasms occur in the vagina, because it contains almost a negligible number of nerve endings. For this reason, a woman may experience her most intense orgasms by the direct stimulation of masturbation or oral sex rather than by intercourse.

The clitoris is a little knob located in the front end of the vulva near the area where a girl urinates. As she and her partner become increasingly sexually excited and intercourse

takes place, she begins to breathe faster, and her breasts en-
large. When she has an orgasm, the vaginal walls near the
opening begin to pulsate rhythmically. After she *comes* her
whole body relaxes. She does not ejaculate fluid as does a
male during orgasm.

During orgasm for a male, semen is ejaculated from
the penis. Muscles around the urethra keep the urine from
coming out with the semen. Just before ejaculation, there are
strong muscular contractions of the penis similar to those in
the female's vaginal walls. After his orgasm, the penis loses
its erection, and the man's whole body relaxes. His breathing
and his blood pressure return to normal, and the sexual flush,
which is a slight reddening of the skin that begins on the
throat and spreads to the stomach, disappears.

Many women never experience an orgasm through sexual
intercourse but find they have a very soothing, satisfying orgasm by means of self-masturbation. When a girl massages her
clitoris she is in complete control of her own sexual release.
She can discover where the most intense sensations around
the clitoris are, she can rub her vulva and clitoris gently,
briskly, slowly, quickly, until she reaches her climax. Masturbation is a very satisfying way for a girl without a sex partner
to have an orgasm. It is a satisfying sexual release after intercourse whenever she has not experienced an orgasm. Masturbation is almost a necessary form of stimulation prior to
intercourse because few men can last the fifteen to twenty-
five minutes it takes for a girl to achieve an orgasm by intercourse.

Sexual response to the point of orgasm is a very healthy
physical release and gives one emotional pleasure and relief
from tensions. Yet it is not good to overemphasize the importance of an orgasm in the success or failure of a sexual
relationship. Many women enjoy sex without an orgasm. The
intimacy, the tenderness, the expression of love that one can
experience in a sexual relationship can give you pleasure
without an orgasm. If you stress having an orgasm too much,
you may not achieve one, for attaining sexual release requires
a full abandonment of one's self just in the enjoyment of the

act of intercourse. It's like happiness—if you chase it too hard, you'll never catch up with it—it will continue to elude you.

Not having an orgasm does not make a girl *less of a woman*, as the old myth goes. An orgasm is something wonderful, pleasurable that happens—but not all the time! It's not necessary to fake or pretend. Tell your partner you enjoy sex with or without an orgasm. Or he can masturbate you to climax so that you will enjoy the emotional satisfaction as well as relief from your tensions.

For those who want, and are unable to have, an orgasm, I would suggest getting advice from a psychiatrist or sex counselor, for the problem is usually psychological.

How can you explain to your parents about your premarital sex?

Why would you want to let your parents know about your premarital sex? What good would it really do? It might alleviate your own guilt, but why put the burden onto someone else? When my son and daughter reached the age of sixteen or older, I assumed they knew what my values were and whether or not they had accepted them. Although, in all honesty, I was curious, I did not expect them to tell me about their sex life. They asked me questions and shared their views about sex, but they did not tell me about their sexual experiences.

Mark expressed the views of several college males I queried when he said: "I feel that you should respect your parents' values and morals on sex, but to let them know that you believe in premarital sex is up to you. My sexual values are based on drawing strict lines of what I think is right and wrong—the same as the basis of my parents'. I feel you can discuss your attitudes about premarital sex with them, but *not* have them know of your experiences with it."

Many of the girls said, "We can't talk about sex at all with our parents—how could we tell them about our sex lives?" Very few felt they could tell their parents about their sexual activities. Betty explained: "It wouldn't be easy. I personally haven't engaged in sex except for serious petting, but if my parents did ask, I would try to be honest and open about it. I wouldn't try to hide the truth because the truth usually comes out—sooner or later. If they have a healthy attitude about sex, they should respect my views. But most of the kids I know have never discussed sexual intercourse or premarital sex at any level with their parents."

Mary believes that you can't really explain to your parents about your premarital sex activity. "When I was sixteen," she said, "I wished they had talked to me about sex, and maybe I might not have gone all the way with a casual friend. Now at eighteen, if they asked me, I would tell them what I think about premarital sex and hope they would respect me, at least, for truthfully telling them how I feel. I wouldn't tell them I am not a virgin, though."

Can the use of marijuana or alcohol affect a person's sex life?

A moderate intake of alcohol can increase the enjoyment of sex by lessening inhibitions. The word *moderate* should be stressed, however. An excessive amount of alcohol can cause the male to become temporarily impotent. Tom, for example, said, "The only time I really want oral sex is when I've been drinking, even though my girl wants me to do it to her very frequently. Of course, when I get too much liquor in me I can't get a hard-on to have sexual intercourse."

Although marijuana and similar drugs contain no sexually stimulating ingredients, some young persons have claimed intensified sexual pleasure, according to psychologists and sexologists. But it is probably only in the mind that drugs increase sexual pleasure. According to research, a continued use of drugs, including marijuana, actually decreases sexual desire and the ability to perform.

Is premarital sex right? Wrong? I guess you will have to decide for yourself, depending upon your own circumstances and maturity. If a boy or girl *under seventeen* asked me this question, however, I would not hesitate to say that I think they are much better off if they avoid sexual intercourse at that age, because this is a deep, meaningful relationship that requires maturity to be properly handled. You might think it is all fun, but it isn't. Fear of discovery, need for concealment, always being in a hurry, risk of venereal disease and pregnancy, take much of the so-called fun out of premarital sex for the young person. The best way to consider premarital sex is to ask yourself if you are prepared to deal with the consequences of this act.

4 venereal disease

ONE MAJOR POTENTIAL EFFECT of sexual intercourse is venereal disease. Judging from the discussions
I've had with college and high-school students, it's clear
that most of you are well aware of venereal disease. Yet
it is continuously on the rise among your age group,
infecting kids even as young as eleven years old. Trag-
ically for the girls, 80 percent of them will have no warning symptoms. The fellows are more fortunate, for the
great majority will have definite indications, such as a
pus discharge from the penis and burning and itching.

How did venereal disease get started anyway?

According to history, the crews of Columbus's ships contracted syphilis in the Caribbean. The disease spread rapidly
throughout Europe during the 1500s after these men brought
the infection back with them. Later, it is believed that when
the Europeans colonized the Americas, they brought the
disease with them. The only real support for this theory is
the recorded fact of a devastating epidemic of syphilis in
Europe during the 1500s.

But where this dreaded disease originated is still a
matter of conjecture. Using the evolutionary theory, sci-
entists suggest that syphilis has evolved from other germs.
It is believed that, in Europe and Asia, so-called *pinta*
germs, which caused a mild skin rash, slowly evolved into
a more serious disease called *yaws*, which could be spread
by body contact through a break in the skin. Syphilis is

thought to have evolved from yaws around 3000 B.C. In early historical accounts, the disease is referred to as *venereal* and *congenital*. Actually, venereal disease of some form or another has probably always existed. And through public ignorance and apathy toward it, syphilis, and gonorrhea in particular, have continued to spread in epidemic proportions.

What kinds of venereal diseases are there? How do I know if I have one?

We have two kinds of diseases that affect the male and female sexual systems—venereal disease—that can be spread only through sexual contact, and nonvenereal disease that can be spread through other means as well. We will talk about the nonvenereal kind first.

Vaginitis is a fairly common inflammation of the vagina. Itching, redness, and soreness, along with a discharge and bad odor, are symptoms. Often young women are overly concerned about keeping themselves clean after sexual intercourse and will use too strong a douche solution. Other causes can be from failing to douche out a contraceptive foam within six to eight hours after intercourse or from leaving a diaphragm in place two or three days at a time. Your doctor will prescribe a five-day treatment with an antibiotic for you and your sexual partner. If your partner is not treated, too, you can continue to reinfect each other. Some types of vaginitis are contacted from the man during intercourse, although he may show no symptoms.

In some cases, a doctor may recommend the use of a mild vinegar douche that will equalize the acid condition of the vagina, which may be upset by the male's semen. It is important for a young woman to use some form of vaginal lubrication such as *K-Y Jelly* before she has sexual intercourse and to be as relaxed as she can. In this way, she can help avoid vaginitis.

Vaginitis can be brought on by sexual tension. Sexual arousal and excitement can be blocked when a girl feels guilt or stress about having intercourse. Without sexual responsiveness, the vaginal lubrication that develops during sexual excitement will not flow, leaving a dry vulva and vagina that can easily be irritated during intercourse.

The best way to avoid vaginitis is to maintain good physical health practices and to develop a positive, healthy attitude toward sex and feminine hygiene. When any discomfort in the genital area develops, one should always consult a doctor immediately. Seeing a gynecologist for a checkup at least once a year is a good idea.

Trichomoniasis is the most common form of genital disease. It can affect both men and women, although men do not suffer the itching, burning, redness, and white or yellowish discharge that women experience. Men have no sign of this disease except a slight watery discharge and perhaps some irritation during urination. This disease is caused by tiny one-celled parasites that limit their attack to the vaginal and penile area. Your doctor will prescribe a medication to be used by *both* partners so that continuing reinfection will not result. Trichomoniasis is most often contracted through intercourse, but it can be picked up in a swimming pool or a bathtub.

Moniliasis, commonly called *Monilia,* is a fungus infection causing inflammation and itching of the genital area. Its symptoms are white cheesy spots on the vulva, in the vagina, and on the cervix of a woman, or under the foreskin of a man's penis. A woman will have a white, watery vaginal discharge, which becomes worse just before and after menstruation. It usually affects women, but children can also pick up this disease from a toilet seat or even a wet towel in a public locker room. It is likely to affect women who have been taking large doses of some antibiotic, which kills off the protective bacilli in the vaginal tract. Pregnant women, those on the Pill, and women who are overweight or diabetic are quite susceptible to this infection. It is essential that both husband and wife be treated for Monilia, particularly since the male acts as a carrier. Unless both are treated and cured, they will continue to reinfect each other. A doctor must be consulted for a prescription to cure this problem, which requires long-term, persistent treatment.

While not a *disease*, the skin irritation caused by *crabs* (tiny parasites also called *pubic lice*) is included in our discussion since crabs are often picked up through sexual contact. They can be picked up also from toilet seats or from trying on bathing suits or underwear others may have worn. That is why it is always wise to wear your underpants when trying on such garments.

The *Crab Louse* will bury its head into the skin and attach itself to the hair follicles. It will spread to all parts of the body where there is hair except the head, biting and causing an itchy skin irritation. When you scratch, further irritation will cause a brownish discoloration of the skin. A druggist can give you the prescribed medication, or you can call the public health department of your city and ask for advice.

Now we will turn to the true venereal diseases: *Herpes* is an acute skin disease caused by a virus. *Herpes Type I* appears as sores on the mouth, or nose. It is generally not sexually transmitted. *Herpes Type II* commonly affects men in the penis and urethra and women in the cervix, vagina, and vulva. It is sexually transmitted through intercourse. Herpes sores at first look like blisters, but they erupt into open sores or ulcers and are very painful. Painful urination is also likely to be experienced by both the man and the woman. The added danger to women is that Herpes II during pregnancy may cause an abortion or premature delivery. The baby may contract the infection from its mother and develop a crippling form of meningitis. Recent evidence indicates that women who have Herpes II are more susceptible to cancer of the cervix. Unfortunately, as yet there is no known safe medical cure for herpes infection.

Pelvic inflammatory disease from rectal sex can have severe repercussions, too. When a man inserts his penis into a woman's rectum for anal intercourse during heavy sex play and then directly goes on to vaginal intercourse, he may transfer various bacteria from the bowel into the woman's pelvic area. This happened to a nineteen-year-old girl recently. She tearfully confided to me that her husband enjoyed rectal sex and they did it often. But as a result, bacteria from her bowel reached her fallopian tubes and there was spillage onto the ovaries. Her whole abdomen became inflamed and she was diagnosed as having appendicitis. Instead, the doctors found that the inflammation she had was so severe that there was no recourse other than surgical removal of her ovaries and fallopian tubes. Here she is at nineteen unable to bear the children she and her husband want.

Another very common bacteria found in the bowel, E. Coli, also can be transferred from the rectum to the woman's urethra when the couple has rectal sex prior to intercourse. This bacteria can cause a serious bladder infection.

Indeed, various bacteria, when transferred from the bowel to the vagina not only can infect the bladder and fallopian tubes, but can also cause cervical bleeding. This is a serious problem particularly since this condition can result from other types of vaginal infections we discussed above. Detection of the bacteria may be difficult unless the girl tells her doctor she has been having rectal sex. She may not reveal this out of embarrassment.

Cleanliness is essential for sex partners. And this is especially true when partners engage in rectal sex. It is *imperative* that a man carefully wash his penis with soap and water after rectal sex before continuing their sex play in any other manner, and especially before he inserts his penis into his partner's vulva and vagina.

Syphilis is the most dangerous of venereal diseases. If it is not cured, it will lead to damage of the vital organs— the heart, liver, kidney, and central nervous system. It can cause blindness, paralysis, heart disease, and insanity.

Syphilis is contracted primarily through sexual intercourse and could be practically avoided by using a condom and washing after intercourse with soap and water. It also can be contacted through kissing or having oral-genital sex with a person who has a syphilitic chancre sore in the mouth or genitalia. It can also be caught by contact of an open scratch with a chancre sore on someone else's body. Telling you the means by which you can get syphilis is not a scare tactic. It is meant only to caution you against intimacy with persons you know very little about.

The chancre is the first sign of syphilis. It is a *painless sore* that appears ten to ninety days after exposure to a person who has this dread disease. The sore is usually found on the penis, anus, or mouth of the male, and in the vagina or mouth of the female. Unfortunately, since it is painless, it may go unnoticed. The most contagious time is within the two-to-four-week period after exposure, but unfortunately, there is no blood test in this early stage that will show it.

Once the disease enters the blood stream, the sore disappears. Then we have the second stage of syphilis, which will present symptoms such as a rash, sore throat, loss of hair, swollen glands, and a run-down feeling. These symptoms can indicate many other mild illnesses, and so the second stage of syphilis often is diagnosed as something else, and the person goes on infecting everyone else with whom he or she has sexual contact, while dooming him or herself to serious consequences. The possibility of undiagnosed syphilis is the main reason why the VDRL blood test (or Wassermann test) is administered before marriage. If this disease has gone undetected, it will be discovered in time to prevent a person from infecting his or her marriage partner.

The third stage of syphilis, which begins one year or more after initial infection, is dangerous because all signs have disappeared and an individual may think that he or she is cured. The fourth stage is very serious as syphilis begins to attack the central nervous system, the heart, the skin, and even the brain. This attack is slow but sure, and about 25 percent of untreated persons become progressively senile. They develop loss of power to concentrate, and other personality disorders such as dullness, irritability, and anxiety. Chronic inflammatory problems may develop involving bones, joints, and eyes.

In addition to the other dangers of syphilis, the fetus of an infected woman will be affected, after fourteen weeks of pregnancy, in the same way as an adult in the third stage. This infant can be born blind or deformed in many other disabling ways, or it may be born dead. But if a mother is treated before the fourth month of pregnancy, the child will usually be born free of the disease.

If you are going to have sexual intercourse with someone you cannot be sure does not have syphilis, why take a chance? A man should have a condom in his pocket and wear it. A woman should insist that her male partner use one. Go to the public health department to find out where you can get a free blood test if you have any reason to believe you have syphilis. The treatment is 2.4 million units of benzathine penicillin. It takes little time or money, and think of the heartache this test and treatment can save.

Gonorrhea is the second most communicable disease next to the common cold, and it can be prevented to a large degree by the use of a condom, and soap and water afterward. It is the leading cause of sterility (the inability to have children) among both men and women. It can also lead to heart disease, crippling arthritis, and blindness. Two to ten days after contacting gonorrhea through sexual intercourse, a person becomes infectious and will pass the disease on to any sex partner. Sex on Thursday, and by Saturday you can infect others.

Men are fortunate in that 80 percent of them will have obvious symptoms such as a burning, itching penis, and a pus discharge from the end of the penis. They may also have swollen glands in the groin and may have pain when they urinate. On the other hand, 80 percent of the women who contact gonorrhea will have no warning symptoms. The few who do may have stomach cramps or pain in urinating for a time, but these go away and meanwhile may be diagnosed as various other minor illnesses, such as a bladder infection.

Usually the only way a girl will know she has gonorrhea is if the man with whom she has had sexual intercourse tells her that he has it. A responsible male will do this, but unfortunately, not all are willing to take this responsibility. As a result, the girl continues to live with this dread disease, which can cause abcesses of her fallopian tubes so that she cannot become pregnant, because the egg cannot pass through to become implanted in her uterus. Babies that are born to mothers with gonorrhea will be born with this disease, resulting in possible blindness and other deformities.

The cure is simple—for a male, a single injection of 2.4 million units of penicillin, and for a female 4.8 million units of penicillin in two injections. It is very important that both partners get treated so that they don't reinfect each other or pass it along to others. Repeated contracting of gonorrhea by the male can have very serious consequences. Every time he gets a new case of gonorrhea, the scar tissues continue to grow up the length of the urethra in his penis. Eventually, the urethra can become completely closed, preventing him from urinating. In order to open up his urethra, the doctor must use an instrument that grinds out the scar tissue. This is very painful and may have limited success. So, gentlemen, beware. Don't think that all there is to a case of gonorrhea is a shot of penicillin. The consequences are far-reaching to you and to those with whom you come in contact sexually.

What should you do if you think you may have venereal disease?

Call the VD Hot Line in your area for the phone number of a venereal disease clinic where you can be tested and then treated if infected. Or call the public health department, which probably has a VD unit, for an appointment, or see your own doctor. And most important, tell your partner immediately so he or she can be tested, too. Remember, the greater number of different sex partners you have, the greater your chance of catching a venereal disease!

Can I have a test for VD or get the cure without my parents finding out?

Yes, in most communities there are free VD clinics, as mentioned above, supported by the Public Health Department, where you can get your shot of penicillin without anyone else knowing about it. If you contact a private doctor, it would be best to ask him about his policy on this before you go see him.

Is it possible to get syphilis or gonorrhea after you are married if neither has had previous experience in sexual intercourse?

No, since these two diseases are contracted primarily through sexual contact—unless, of course, one of you has had oral sex with someone who had syphilis.

As stated earlier, the blood test required in all states prior to marriage detects syphilis. It is also important to ask the doctor or clinic to give you a test for gonorrhea prior to marriage if you have been sexually active. Responsible behavior on the part of all sexually active people in reporting their suspicions of VD and seeking treatment is the only way we are going to wipe out this terrible affliction.

How can I be free of VD but remain sexually active?

Prevention is the key word when considering venereal diseases. Unfortunately preventing VD is very difficult for many reasons. While more young people are becoming sexually active, many are irresponsible about their own health, the health of their sex partners, or the prevention of a premarital pregnancy. With the availability of other forms of birth control methods (even though research indicates that young people are not using them) the condom, which offers good protection against venereal disease and pregnancy, is not being used to the extent it should.

Education has failed to get across the hazards to your health that promiscuous sexual behavior can have, particularly with respect to the dreadful consequences of venereal disease that goes untreated. Oftentimes, persons who contract VD are youngsters who come from unhappy homes where they have been caused to feel themselves unloved or worthless. They think they will find a boost to their sense of worth through many sexual contacts. Sex will not solve emotional problems. It can create problems—emotional, social, and physical.

VD is everywhere—it is contracted by all kinds of people in all parts of our society. It will not be prevented until people learn the importance of keeping their bodies healthy and clean. Think enough of yourself to protect your body from VD. Become aware of how your body works and of the responsibility you have to prevent venereal disease.

5 preventing pregnancy

JUDGING FROM THE MANY QUESTIONS asked me about birth control, it's clear that teenagers are very interested in the subject. Yet despite the ready availability of many different types of contraceptives, many of you do not use them during intercourse. Why not? Perhaps you do not think pregnancy is something that can happen to *you*.

Planned Parenthood reports that 30 percent of sexually active teenage girls become pregnant. The fact is that one girl in ten is a mother before she reaches her eighteenth birthday. A teenager's baby is three times as likely to die before its first birthday than a baby born to a mother who is twenty. A teenager's baby is more likely to have birth defects such as spinal injury, breathing problems, mental retardation, and clubfoot. The teenage mother is destined to become a high-school dropout; in fact, eight out of ten pregnant teenagers under age seventeen do not finish school. If she marries the father, chances of a divorce are more than double those of girls who wait to marry and to have a child until after they are twenty-two.

A teenage pregnancy hurts everyone—the babies whose life chances are smaller; the mother who must cope with all the problems of parenthood when she is still often a child herself. Pregnancy for a teenager can be so depressing that research shows seven times as many pregnant school-age mothers commit suicide as do girls who have never been pregnant. The father may be financially strapped or feel forced to marry his child's mother. The grandparents, who often are unwilling, must share the raising of an unwanted or unplanned-for child. The taxpayers pay the cost of welfare for many teenage mothers and their babies. Studies show that 60 percent of all teenage mothers are supported by welfare.

Two-thirds of all teenage pregnancies are unintended. If you haven't been concerned about birth control until now, you had better start taking it seriously if you plan to remain sexually active.

What is birth control and what type would you recommend for an unmarried seventeen-year-old girl like myself?

Birth control means doing something to prevent either conception or the birth of a child. There are three main methods of birth control: abstinence, sterilization, and contraception.

Abstinence means that a person does not engage in sexual intercourse at all. This person may take care of his or her sexual desires through masturbation or petting to orgasm.

Sterilization means that a man or woman is made sterile, that is, becomes unable to produce a child when they do have sexual intercourse. Women may become sterilized in several ways. However, sterilization is *not* recommended for young women who may want to have children in the future, though there is a form of *reversible sterilization* available. This method involves the doctor's placing small clips around the fallopian tubes so that the sperm is blocked from reaching the egg. When a woman wants to become pregnant, the doctor, through a certain procedure, can remove the clips. While this procedure is quite successful in restoring the probability of a woman's being able to conceive a child, restoration is only between 25 and 50 percent.

Other forms of sterilization include a *tubal ligation*, which involves major surgery to cut and tie the fallopian tubes so the two ends can't meet, thus preventing sperm from getting through to the egg. This is a form of *permanent sterilization.*

Another means of closing the fallopian tubes involves cauterizing the ends. This is done by making two tiny punctures in the abdomen and inserting an electrical cauterizing instrument.

A type of sterilization that many of you have probably heard about is a *hysterectomy.* This involves the surgical removal of the uterus and may also include removal of the ovaries and fallopian tubes. This method is also permanent. It is done to correct abnormalities or malignancies and not as an elective method of sterilization.

Sterilization is not recommended by many doctors except when it is quite certain that the mother has a hereditary disorder or a medical problem that would cause her to bear a defective child, or when bearing children might cause the mother's death. Even in matters of a mother's health, a doctor may have legal problems. Written consent by the patient cannot prevent a suit's being filed against a doctor in most states.

If a couple is considering sterilization, it seems that a *vasectomy* for the male would be the wisest choice. In recent years this method of sterilization has become more and more popular in our society. Perhaps this is due in part to the fact that sterilization for a man has fewer complications than for a woman. A *vasectomy* can usually be done in about twenty minutes in a doctor's office or on an outpatient basis under a local anesthetic in a hospital. It is far less expensive than is sterilization for a woman because it is not major surgery requiring hospitalization, as are most types of sterilization for women.

A vasectomy involves cutting and tying the duct, known as the vas deferens, that carries the sperm. When the duct is tied, the sperm cannot pass from the testicles to the ejaculatory duct during intercourse. The man remains perfectly able to have sex, but he cannot cause a woman to become pregnant. There is over a 60 percent chance that vasectomies can be reversed by surgically rejoining the ends of the vas deferens. This is an important consideration for a young man who may marry the second time and whose new wife may want children, or for a couple who may decide at a later date they want to start having children to add to their family. There is also a small chance that a vasectomy may be unsuccessful and pregnancy may result. It is important that the man have about twenty to thirty ejaculations before he can be sure he is sterile. He should be tested twice for sperm-free semen before he makes this assumption. Until then, the birth control previously used should be continued. I think that a vasectomy is a very effective method of birth control and allows the man to take the responsibility for not getting a woman pregnant. It does not affect his ability to perform or his enjoyment of sex. Reports indicate that it may actually increase his sex drive.[1] It is hoped that this type of birth control will continue to increase among married couples after they have the children they desire. Reversing a vasectomy is becoming more likely as newer and more successful methods of reversal are being achieved.

   Contraception refers to any method of preventing pregnancy during sexual intercourse. Included in types of contraceptives are the *condom*, the *diaphragm*, the *oral contraceptive pill*, and the *intrauterine contraceptive device*, known as the IUD. The first three are best suited for use by unmarried persons.

What are the benefits of using a condom?

A condom is readily available, easily disposable, relatively inexpensive and, as we have said, is a good protection against both venereal disease and pregnancy when properly used. The pregnancy rate of the condom averages about 10 or 11, although the range is from 6 to 19, depending upon the precautions taken with its use.* It is also a method that allows the male to assume responsibility for protection against an unwanted pregnancy.

---

*A pregnancy rate of 10 means that couples using condoms had 10 pregnancies per 100 years. Pregnancy rates are determined by a formula that considers the number of pregnancies that occur to a certain number of persons over a certain period of years. For example, if 50 pregnancies occur to 100 couples during a 5-year period, the pregnancy rate would be 10. The formula reads:

$$\text{pregnancy rate} = \frac{\text{number of pregnancies} \times \text{years}}{\text{patients observed} \times \text{years of exposure}} = \frac{50 \times 100}{100 \times 5} = \frac{5000}{500} = 10$$

A rate under 10 is very high in effectiveness. A rate between 10 and 20 is medium, according to N. J. Eastman and L. Hellman in their book, *Williams Obstetrics* (New York: Appleton, 1961).

When unrolled, the condom looks like a deflated balloon about seven and one-half inches long, with a diameter of one and a half inches. Most condoms are made of a thin, strong latex rubber; some are made from sterile animal gut membrane. Rubber condoms are the most popular because they are cheaper and just as effective as the skin condoms.

The condom is fastened to a narrow rubber ring. To put on a condom, the man places the ring on the tip of his erect penis; he then unrolls the condom onto his penis. The condom should be unrolled one-half inch before it is unrolled over the penis, however. This small excess tip will receive the semen when the man ejaculates. The half-inch space left at the end of the condom should be squeezed while putting it on so that air is not trapped inside it. If a man is not circumcised, he should pull back the foreskin before unrolling the condom onto his penis.

To make inserting the penis into the girl's vagina pleasant and easy, I suggest that she lubricate herself by inserting an applicator full of a spermicidal cream or jelly into her vagina, which also gives an additional contraceptive protection. Or the man can use a prelubricated condom or rub some surgical jelly over the condom after it is rolled on. But never use vaseline or any kind of petroleum jelly, for it will destroy rubber!

The problems with using condoms are breakage during use (which seldom happens) and having the condom slip off during withdrawal, which may allow semen to get into the girl's vagina. If care is taken in pulling out after ejaculation, the condom is unlikely to slip off. The man should always hold on to the condom at the base of his penis during withdrawal to prevent it from slipping off. Should the condom break, the use of spermicidal jelly or cream, as suggested above, will reduce the chances of pregnancy. As an added precaution, the girl should insert an applicator full of the spermicidal jelly or cream into her vagina immediately after intercourse if breakage has occurred or the condom has slipped off the penis. To make certain of high-quality condoms, purchase them only from drugstores or family-planning agencies; no prescription is necessary. Those obtained in men's washrooms are likely to be of poor quality.

If the condom is so simple to use and readily available, why aren't more young people using it?

I have heard of three *excuses*. According to the *myth* spread by some young men, using a condom takes away some of a man's pleasure of feeling his penis inside a woman's vagina. Actually, this cannot be, for condoms are extremely thin and transmit *feelings* very well. It certainly allows him to have an orgasm, and this is probably the most pleasurable feeling a man gets. The objection that putting on a condom interrupts the spontaneity of lovemaking can be overcome by including the act of rolling the condom onto her lover's penis as the girl's part of the love play.

The third reason given me for not using a condom is that girls get angry when a man pulls one out of his pocket. "You cad, you intended to do this to me when you asked me for a date! What kind of a girl do you think I am?" is the response several young men tell me they have received. Of course, in this case, a man can tell his date that he just likes to assume responsibility for his own welfare as well as his date's in case things do turn out this way. That ought to modify a girl's attitudes, and if it doesn't, shouldn't he forget about intercourse at that particular time? Actually, men who refuse to use a condom because of these reasons are just copping out from their responsibility.

What about the Pill?

One of the most popular contraceptives, and certainly the most effective form of preventing conception is the Pill. From present research, I feel confident that it is *relatively* safe, although it is important to emphasize that long-term effects of taking the Pill are still unknown. The many questions asked about it indicate that there is considerable concern about its use. Certainly most of the studies I have read indicate that the use of oral contraceptives under the direction of a doctor has proved to be safe for most women.

I am under eighteen. Can I get the Pill without my parents' consent?

According to the U.S. Supreme Court Rulings, age is no barrier to obtaining contraceptives without parental consent. Druggists and family-planning clinics are free to dispense certain forms of contraceptives without parental consent, and for some (such as condoms, creams, and jellies), without a prescription from a doctor. But there is no law forcing a doctor or a druggist to make them available to a minor.

What is the Pill made of and how does it work?

The birth control pill is made of synthetic hormones called progesterone and estrogen which, when taken, prevent ovulation of the egg. When no egg or ovum is released, no pregnancy can occur. There are a variety of combinations of synthetic hormones in various dosages and strengths. The doctor, after a careful physical examination, will decide upon the proper prescription for a woman. If side effects (which we shall discuss later) don't subside, the physician will change the prescription when the problem is reported to him.

How do I take the Pill?

After a doctor makes the birth control pill available to you, you would begin taking it on the fifth day from the beginning of your monthly menstrual period. At the same hour each day, you should take one pill for exactly twenty days, or twenty-one days, depending upon the directions from the doctor. Your next menstrual period will begin from two to five days after taking the last pill. You must not skip a pill, for although the chance of getting pregnant is remote, there is a possibility of pregnancy. Some girls *share* their pills with their friends, but this can be dangerous to girls who have not been examined by a doctor to make sure it is safe for them to take it. And, of course, taking a pill now and then will not prevent pregnancy, so *don't share yours with your friends.*

Do I have to have a physical before I can get the Pill? What happens during a physical?

Yes, you do need to have a physical examination.

The *physical exam* begins with the doctor's asking you questions about your menstrual cycle, any illnesses you have had, and, if you say you have been sexually active, what birth control methods you have used. Next, after you have completely undressed, the nurse gives you a disposable gown to put on. The nurse will then take your blood pressure, weigh you, and measure your height. She will also take a blood sample and ask you to leave a urine specimen. When the doctor returns, you will be sitting on the examining table, and he or she will examine your neck, your chest, back, lungs, heart, and stomach area. Then, you will be asked to lie down and put your legs in two stirrup-like supports so that your legs will be kept apart while the doctor examines your vaginal area. You won't feel too embarrassed because you will have a sheet over your body with only the vaginal area exposed. The doctor will most likely talk to you during your exam to put you at ease. Remember, to the doctor, you are a *patient,* and there is nothing *sexy* about this exposure.

The first thing the doctor will do is put an instrument, called a speculum, into your vagina (this will feel cold at first) to spread and hold apart the vaginal walls. While your vagina is spread, the doctor will insert an instrument to gently scrape some tissue from your cervix for a Pap smear, a routine test that detects cervical cancer. This test feels the way it would if someone gently scratched your hand with a fingernail. The doctor will then take out the instruments and, with his or her gloved hand, will give you an *internal* examination by inserting two fingers into your vagina. The doctor's other hand will press down on your lower abdomen to feel your uterus and other reproductive organs. If there are any problems, they will be indicated by this internal exam, along with the other exam and test. After examining you thoroughly, the doctor will be in a position to recommend a contraceptive for you.

Unfortunately, many girls do not seek contraceptives when becoming sexually active because of the embarrassment they feel about the prospect of having a vaginal exam. Parents generally neglect their young daughters' sexual health. Thus, many girls are totally ignorant about their bodies. Young girls are subject to cervical cancer, as well as breast cancer, and therefore should have regular physical exams to detect these problems.

Many girls are embarrassed about going to a male doctor for what is probably their first vaginal and pelvic examination. There are many female gynecologists available and very often the person who will give the examination in a family-planning or other public health clinic will be a female. If you feel funny about going to a male doctor, check with the local medical association or Public Health Department for names of female physicians.

I have heard that the Pill is unsafe for a woman's health. Is it really harmful?

From the research I have read, I feel confident to say that, when used as instructed, the Pill is relatively safe. When taken as directed, the resultant pregnancy rate is only 0.10, making it the most effective contraceptive there is. When a woman wants to become pregnant, all she has to do is quit using the Pill and, eventually, usually within a year or less, she will become pregnant if she is normally fertile. In terms of the Pill's potential danger, research tells us that the risk of dying from childbirth is far greater than from the Pill.[2] However, before using it, it is important to consider other effective forms of contraceptives that have been around longer, and whose long-term effects are clearly known.

I have heard there are some side effects when taking the Pill. What are they?

Side effects are most often minor and are usually psychological in nature. That is, if you expect certain side effects, they may very well appear. A mild form of nausea, sometimes involving vomiting or stomach cramps, is the most common side effect. This can be avoided by taking the Pill on a full stomach or with a glass of milk right before going to bed.

A general bloated feeling, breast discomfort, quick weight gain, or itching of the skin can accompany *fluid retention* because of the estrogen in the Pill. If severe headaches or dizziness accompanies this water retention, then the doctor will probably recommend that you stop taking the Pill or change the dosage. Water retention does not happen frequently, and it can be lessened by a low-salt diet.

Other possible side effects, which seldom happen, include depression and lessening of sexual desire, enlargement of breasts, fatigue, oily skin and hair. If a girl experiences these problems, she should see her doctor so that he can change the prescription. There are many combinations of estrogen and progesterone hormones, and the doctor usually can find one for you that will eliminate these side effects.

One does hear about serious side effects resulting from the Pill. There have been reports about complications such as a blood clot's forming in a blood vessel, preventing the flow of blood in the body. This condition is known as *thromboembolism*. It does not occur often, however. Of course, every drug carries some risk to its user. If you smoke or consume alcoholic beverages, you are running much, much graver risks to your health than you would by taking the Pill. You should be cautioned that girls who smoke or who are overweight should not use the Pill because they are likely to have the above complications. The Pill may entail some risk, but it is the *surest* contraceptive aside from abstinence. Before you decide to become sexually active, discuss with your doctor any concerns or questions you have about the Pill.

What about the diaphragm?

Another form of birth control rising in popularity is the *diaphragm*. The diaphragm is a smooth rubber cup fastened onto a rubber-covered metal ring. It looks like a little dome and is constructed so that it fits over the mouth of the cervix to prevent semen and sperm from entering the uterus. Before it is used, the girl places in the diaphragm some spermicidal jelly or cream that serves as a lubricant as well as an added protection against pregnancy.

You can only get a diaphragm by prescription from a doctor or from a family-planning clinician, such as those in the Planned Parenthood organization. Each woman's body is different, so it is necessary that the diaphragm be fitted to each woman's particular size. After the correct size and shape is determined, the doctor will show you how to insert the diaphragm so that it covers the cervix correctly. This is not very complicated. You simply slide the diaphragm up into your vagina as far as it can go. You can feel with your finger if it is in place so that it covers the cervix. Your gynecologist will make certain you can do this properly.

After a girl has had sexual intercourse, she should not remove the diaphragm for at least six hours, and it can be left in for as long as twenty-five hours without any discomfort. In order to remove the diaphragm, the girl just has to hook her finger under the ring and gently pull it down and out. This only takes a second or two. The diaphragm should be checked occasionally by filling it with water to make sure there is no seepage.

Although the diaphragm with spermicidal foam, cream, or jelly is almost as effective in preventing pregnancy as the birth control pill, one often hears the complaint that it interferes with the spontaneity that makes intercourse enjoyable. This is ridiculous, for if you know that intercourse is likely, all you have to do is insert the diaphragm as part of your nightly ritual. It takes no longer than brushing your teeth, and if you do have intercourse, you are ready; if not, it only takes a few seconds in the morning to remove the diaphragm.

If a girl has not had sexual intercourse, a doctor usually will not recommend a diaphragm, for she cannot be fitted until after her hymen is broken. If a physician or family-planning clinician does fit her with a diaphragm, she will have to be checked again after intercourse, because her vagina will be stretched and she may need to be refitted. Generally, with proper use, a diaphragm plus jelly or cream is a very effective contraceptive with no known side effects.

The pregnancy rate is 4 to 10 for the diaphragm when used properly. The spermicidal jelly or cream is effective for two hours, so if repeated intercourse takes place, the girl should insert an applicator full of the jelly or cream into her vagina prior to making love again.

What is an IUD?

The *intrauterine contraceptive device*, or *IUD*, is a small, plastic device designed to fit into the uterus. It comes in various shapes—spiral, loop, ring, bow, or T.

Many doctors do not recommend an IUD for a woman who has not been pregnant or who has not given birth to a child. The smaller, tighter uterus of a girl who has not been pregnant may cause her to feel pain during and immediately after insertion. She may also feel cramps and bleeding for the first few days after insertion. Sometimes the pain is so severe that immediate removal by the doctor becomes necessary. The IUD, then, is recommended primarily for women who have already been pregnant and who are over thirty years of age.

The IUD prevents implantation in the uterine wall of the egg or ovum after it is fertilized by the male sperm. Pregnancy, thus, cannot occur. This device can only be obtained through a prescription written by a physician, who must fit it into the uterus. The insertion of an IUD is usually a quick, simple, and relatively painless procedure. Before a woman is fitted, the doctor will make a general examination of her vaginal and pelvic areas. He or she will also take a Pap test. The IUD is placed in the uterine cavity, leaving two nylon

threads that are connected to the device and hang down into
the upper vagina. The threads are trimmed so that about two
inches remain below the cervix. They can easily be felt, and a
woman wearing the IUD should check herself frequently to
make sure it has not become dislodged. Most expulsions
occur within the first three or four months after the device
is in the uterus. This usually happens during the menstrual
period, so women using an IUD should *always* check the sur-
face of their menstrual pads or tampons to ensure it has not
become dislodged.

The best time to have an IUD inserted is on the first day
of a menstrual period to be sure that you are not already
pregnant. Also, insertion of the IUD may cause a slight
amount of bleeding from the uterus, and this will not be an
additional problem during menstruation.

The IUD, with a pregnancy rate of 2 to 3, is a very
effective contraceptive for those who can use it. It is also
safe, with a few exceptions that happen very infrequently,
according to McCary.[3] Sometimes the device fails to remain in the uterus and goes through the uterine wall into
the abdominal cavity. Such perforations usually require
immediate surgery to correct the problem.

Should a girl become pregnant with the device still in
place, there is usually no danger to the baby. It is removed
when the baby is born. In recent years, there was one type of
IUD that caused serious bleeding and sometimes the death
of the woman or a spontaneous aborting of the fetus when
pregnancy occurred. This type has since been taken off the
market, and no further cases have occurred, to my knowledge. On the basis of available studies, uterine or cervical
cancer is not caused by the use of an IUD, contrary to some
old wives' tales. The IUD should remain in place until the
woman wishes to become pregnant. Then she must have the
doctor remove it, and after she has a child, another IUD may
be inserted. It is important to stress that *under no circumstances should* a woman attempt to remove the IUD by herself, for serious bleeding and other complications, such as
infection, could occur.

Are there any other means of contraception?

Contraceptive foam is effective if it is injected deep inside the vagina no earlier than fifteen to thirty minutes prior to intercourse. It will block the sperm from entering the cervix, and it also has a toxic action against sperm. One objection to foam is that it is messy when the couple is involved in love play. If you wait until after the foreplay, there will be an interruption to inject the foam. (Of course injecting the foam into the girl's vagina could become part of the sex play.) Messy as foam is, it cannot be douched out for at least eight hours after ejaculation. The pregnancy rate of spermicidal foams ranges from about 6 to 27, indicating that failure rate can be pretty high. Delfen and Emko brands are the most effective foams. Directions must be followed very carefully in order for the foam to be effective in preventing conception. However, the foam is far better than using no protection.

Spermicidal creams and *jellies* are not very effective by themselves. However, as I mentioned earlier, when used with condoms or the diaphragm, they are very effective.

Douches must not be considered a means of preventing conception. The sperm move so quickly into the uterus that a douche is too late; rather, it might help speed the sperm upward to the cervix. Don't ever believe the myth that douching with a cola drink is in any way a birth control method.

There are a couple of other types of birth control that people use with a remarkable degree of *unsuccess.* I am speaking of *withdrawal* and the *Rhythm Method.*

Withdrawal has many disadvantages. A man cannot really relax and enjoy sexual intercourse when he has to be on the alert to pull out just before he *comes.* This is not good for the girl either, for under the strain, she may not be able to relax sufficiently to enjoy sex or have an orgasm. In addition, the risk of pregnancy is always present when a couple relies on withdrawal. Sperm cells are present in the secretion from the penis during arousal, so that a pregnancy can occur even though the man does not ejaculate. If he is slow to withdraw, just a drop of semen contains many sperm.

The *Rhythm Method* depends upon a couple having sex during the few days when the girl is not supposed to be able to conceive. The problem is that it is very difficult to predict accurately when this period may happen. A bad cold, an emotional upset, or unusual excitement may upset the cycle so that ovulation changes its time. If a woman does not have regular menstrual periods, it is almost impossible for her to predict precisely the safe period. Research tells us that very few women have a period regular enough to count on the Rhythm Method.

The important factor in successfully using any form of birth control is proper knowledge of how it should be used. Young people between the ages of ten and seventeen are notably lacking in adequate information about these methods of preventing the birth of a child that is unplanned or unwanted.

If you feel you are mature enough to enter into a relationship that includes sexual intercourse, one clear indication is the willingness to take on the responsibility of birth control. After you read the next chapter, titled "Single and Pregnant," I hope you will realize more than ever that using an effective contraceptive, if you are sexually active, is of vital importance, particularly for your own social and psychological well-being. A premarital pregnancy is a tragedy for most teenagers, and even more tragic is the fact that it could so easily be prevented with responsible sexual behavior.

6 single and pregnant

"BUT WHAT IF I become pregnant?" is a question apparently seldom considered by many teenagers who decide to become sexually active. After all, more than one million teenagers become pregnant each year. According to the *Wall Street Journal*, there were 447,900 illegitimate births in 1975 (the latest figure available).[1] Sixty percent of all unwed mothers are teenagers.[2] In other words, in 1975, there were 268,740 unwed teenage mothers. Each year this number increases, and the number of pregnant girls between the ages of thirteen to fifteen is rising the most rapidly in our society. In fact, 30,000 girls younger than fifteen get pregnant each year.[3]

Why are so many teenagers becoming pregnant? Part of the reason, as we have seen, is that many of you don't want to be bothered about the responsibility of birth control. Others are simply ignorant about the whole process of reproduction, not really associating sex with pregnancy. Some girls think they are in love and believe that having a child is the *romantic* thing to do. Many girls are so starved for love that they wrongly believe a baby can give them the affection they want. But, in fact, no one really knows the exact reason a girl and boy have an illegitimate child. I hope that the following questions and answers will alleviate some of the false notions and lack of information that many of you may have about having or not having babies.

When can a girl become pregnant?

A girl is physically developed enough to become pregnant when she begins to menstruate. This can happen anytime between the ages of nine and seventeen. The menstrual period lasts three to seven days. Then about fourteen or fifteen days after the *beginning* of the period, ovulation takes place. Ovulation is the release of an egg or ovum from the ovaries. From the moment of ovulation and for about ten more days, a girl can become pregnant. When a couple has sexual intercourse during this period, the sperm can quickly find its way up into the fallopian tube where the egg goes after it leaves the ovary. If a sperm from the male's ejaculation of semen penetrates the egg, *fertilization* has taken place. About six days after fertilization, the egg will attach itself to the inside walls of the uterus, and if it successfully implants itself and begins to thrive, we can say that *conception* has taken place. If implantation does not occur, then the girl will menstruate again at her regular time.

What are the signs of being pregnant?

The most usual sign of pregnancy is a late menstrual period. If a girl is ten days late, she can be considered about thirty-five days pregnant, since pregnancy is figured from the first day of the last menstrual period. Of course, being late for a period can be due to illness, some emotional disturbance, and the like. So, if a woman wants to know for sure, she must see her doctor or a family-planning clinic for an examination and tests.

When a girl is two weeks overdue and has reason to believe she is pregnant, she can request a urine test, receiving the results in about six hours. Her urine is injected into a rat or rabbit, and if the girl is pregnant, the injection causes a reaction, such as ovulation, in the animal. Another pregnancy test can be made, in which a chemical is added to the urine and a particular chemical reaction shows whether or not the woman is pregnant. This test only takes about fifteen or twenty minutes.

A vial containing a chemical to use in a new early pregnancy test (E.P.T.) can be purchased at drugstores. The test involves mixing the chemical with the first urine sample of the morning. You let this mixture of chemical and urine sit *undisturbed* for two hours. If you are pregnant, you will see a dark brown doughnut-shaped ring in the bottom center of the vial.

All of these tests are generally accurate, but a girl should also go to a doctor for confirmation. She will receive a pelvic examination similar to the one described in the preceding chapter on birth control. The doctor can determine if a pregnancy exists if the cervix is softer than usual and if the uterus has become enlarged. Other signs of pregnancy include swollen or tender breasts, more frequent urination, constipation, fatigue, and *morning sickness* or nausea.

Can a doctor or clinic give you a pregnancy test when you are under eighteen without your parents knowing or without the doctor prying?

The family-planning clinic in your area will give you a pregnancy test without asking you any questions about your age or marital status. Whether a doctor will do this without asking you questions or telling your parents is strictly up to the doctor. The thing to do is to inquire first about the physician's policies in this matter before you make an appointment.

Is it true that you can have your period three months after you've had sexual intercourse and be pregnant?

You would not have a regular full menstrual period at this time, but it is possible to have a few days of bleeding, which might mean that there is a possibility of a miscarriage. This means that the fetus will be expelled from your body, and you will no longer be pregnant. In any case, it would be very wise to go immediately to a doctor or clinic for an examination and advice. Often the bleeding will stop as it started, with your pregnancy remaining intact.

What choices do an unwed boy and girl have when a pregnancy happens?

The unwed couple has four alternatives. The girl can keep the child as a single parent; she can give it up for adoption; she can have an abortion; or the couple can get married. None of these alternatives is simple or easy to choose. All of them have to be evaluated rationally. What are your long-range goals for your life? Did you want a career, college? You will probably need help in making your decision, and it is very important to be able to talk to someone about it—lover, friend, doctor, parents, clergy.

If I were pregnant, I would want to keep my baby even though I had no intention of marrying its father. What kinds of problems does a single mother face?

Over 90 percent of unmarried teenage girls who bear children keep them. I consider this to be very unfortunate. Not only are these mothers usually too immature to assume the responsibilities of parenthood, but they also have very little understanding of what it can mean to head a single-parent family. If they decide to live away from their own parents, they are apt to find themselves in a poor financial situation and may have to live on welfare. They may be forced to live in poor housing in bad neighborhoods because of their poverty. If they have little money, they will have less than adequate diets and receive little medical attention for themselves or their babies. Caring for a baby takes patience and time, and when a teenage mother attempts childcare alone without the support that a husband could give, she may become very frustrated and unhappy. The father does have legal responsibilities for support until the child is eighteen, but often the teenage mother will not, or cannot, identify the father. The father may deny the child is his, and it is very difficult to prove paternity. Single parenthood is not an altogether pleasant choice, particularly for the baby, even when this decision has the support of the mother's parents.

Why, then, do so many young girls opt for single parent-hood?

Initially, a teenager thinks about keeping her baby because of outside pressure to do so. Her school friends are very likely to encourage her to keep the baby. "Won't it be fun to have a sweet, cuddly baby to love?" they say to this pregnant girl. So she may keep the child because it seems so right. But after the baby arrives and the reality of childcare and respon-sibility hits home—feeding, diapering, losing sleep when the baby wakes at night, losing freedom to go out with her friends because the baby needs constant care—she realizes that a baby is much more than a cuddly toy. Often the girl is unable to complete her high-school or college education. As Jeanie, a former student of mine, said, "My mother told me I could keep the baby, and she would help me take care of it. But now the baby is here, and she has decided to take a job outside the home, so I am trapped with taking care of the baby and doing all the housework and cooking, too. I'll never get back to school now."

Marge, an eighteen-year-old mother, came to me for ad-vice after two years of living on welfare and trying to care for her child. "I am afraid I am really going to hurt my son se-riously," she said. "I just can't stand his crying, and spanking him never makes him stop. Why did I let those so-called friends of mine talk me into keeping it? After the baby came, they deserted me as if I had something catching. I can't take my kid on dates, and my mother thinks I am terrible because she found out I went out and left the baby alone for several hours. But what's a girl going to do? I can't stay penned up in that lousy apartment all the time."

Marge is quite typical of the young girls who decide to keep their babies, remain single, and live by themselves. They have very little income, little education; they tend to blame their plight on the innocent child; due to their resentment, they are potential child abusers, as we will discuss later.

Jill is glad she kept her baby, but she has problems, too. "My boyfriend is seventeen and has not graduated from high school, and I am a freshman in college. My parents and his parents told me if I kept the baby, they would both help so I can continue in college. His mother takes care of my six-month-old daughter afternoons when I am in school, but she is always giving me digs about kids who are so dumb to get caught. My parents are always reminding me of how they thought they would be free from taking care of kids when I graduated from school, and now they will probably be stuck for a long time. My mother, especially, is very embarrassed about my having a baby and reminds me often of our social disgrace. Dad is always saying, 'Where did we go wrong?' But I do appreciate the help my parents and his parents are giving me. They really are nice about it. They really love little Amy. I worry about the future, though. And I don't want to marry this guy because he's just not my type. I would never give my baby to anyone—I love her.''

Girls who are eighteen or over, who may have a job, savings, and an apartment when they become pregnant, may not have as many problems as the younger girl. With the aid of welfare, if necessary, they may be able to provide adequate, loving care and shelter for the child they decide to keep. Regardless of an unwed mother's age or circumstances, however, keeping her child is usually beset with problems. When she lives by herself with her child she faces all the same difficulties of other women heading single-parent families. Being young, she may have quit school and not have sufficient education or training to support herself and her baby adequately. Finances, finding a job, loneliness, finding someone to care for her child if she works, or in the evenings if she wants to go out, and dating are all problems for a single parent. And these problems are often worse than usual because of her status as unwed. Will guys think she is an "easy lay" because she is a single parent? Will they be interested in her as a potential mate when marriage would mean taking on the responsibilities of another man's child?

These various difficulties will be discussed in greater detail later on in this chapter.

What about adoption?

Giving her child up for adoption is often less problematic for the single mother, and it may be much better for the baby to go into a stable home with two loving parents. The main blocks to adoption are emotional. Girls have said to me, "I could never carry a baby inside of me for nine months, and then give it up to someone else." I can appreciate how very difficult this decision would be to make, but it has been done successfully by many girls, though seldom easily. Girls who decide to give up their baby for adoption rarely ever see their baby to hold or feed. In this way, the separation is said to be less traumatic. The thought that adoption is best for the baby's well-being is consolation, but nothing heals the loss that some girls feel except time.

I have counseled girls who have released their children for adoption and who now wonder if they made the right decision. I encourage them to think about the loving home their child has with a mother and a father who wanted a baby so much that there could be little doubt that the baby was receiving all the care it could need. Then I ask them to think about what they could have given their baby had they kept it.

Joan, a college freshman, gave up her baby for adoption and she explained her experience to me: "It was difficult to decide after I had had it in my body for nine months. But I knew I was not ready or willing to be a mother at the age of seventeen. If I had kept the baby, I would not be in college right now. But I can tell you, right before I signed the final papers, I almost backed down. I am glad now I didn't. I feel a terrible loss, though, and I know I probably will never forget about having had that baby. The good thing is that I know he has a very good life now with a mother and father who really love him and will give him the advantages of a really good home, which I could never do. It's hard on me emotionally, but looking at the girls I know who kept their babies, I am really much better off."

Betty, a nineteen-year-old college freshman, gave up her son for adoption when she was fifteen. "I had no other choice, for I could not get married to a fifteen-year-old boy, and my parents couldn't afford to keep a baby for me," she explained. "Mother, Dad, our doctor, and our minister were very helpful to me. They didn't condemn me, but they made me understand that my whole future would be better if I gave up my baby to some people who couldn't have a child of their own. My mother was also concerned about what people would say about me and her and Dad, too. They didn't want my younger brothers and sisters to know either. So they sent me out to visit my aunt in Colorado, explaining to everyone that, perhaps, a change in climate would help alleviate my *asthma*. When I came back a year later, no one knew what had really happened to me except my parents, doctor, and minister. But *I* knew what had happened! Even after four years, whenever I see a little blond, blue-eyed boy who looks like the father of my child, I want to run to him and pick him up and kiss him. I often wonder where my baby is and what he is like. I'll probably never stop wondering. Still, I believe I did the right thing for my baby and for myself and family. I wouldn't want to be a bad influence on my four younger sisters, either."

I promised to make no value judgments about anyone's choice regarding sexual behavior, but let me have one little bias. I want to urge teenagers who have decided to take the risk of becoming parents by having sexual intercourse out of wedlock to think through very carefully what they would do if a pregnancy occurred. Unless you are planning to get married in the future, really love each other, or have loving parents who will be willing to care for your child until you are socially and emotionally ready to take over the responsibility, adoption is probably the right answer. Unfortunately, only about six percent of teenage mothers give up their babies for adoption, according to recent reports.[4]

What happens when you have an abortion?

The alternative chosen by almost half of all teenage girls who become pregnant out of wedlock is *abortion*. Abortion is the induced expulsion of a fetus from the uterus before it has developed sufficiently to survive outside the mother. The simplest, low-cost abortion is the *vacuum* or *suction* method, but it must be done within two or three weeks after the first missed period. This means that as soon as a girl suspects she may be pregnant she must consider abortion, if that is what she intends to do about her pregnancy. In this method of abortion, the cervical canal is opened and a tube is inserted into the uterus so that a vacuum pump can suck out the embryo. The procedure can be done in a doctor's office with very little pain involved.

If the pregnancy has not gone beyond the twelfth week, a method of abortion called *dilation and curettage* (a *"d & c"*) may be done. This procedure is done in the hospital under an anesthetic. The cervical canal is opened to allow a spoonlike instrument, called a curette, to be inserted into the uterus. Using this instrument, the doctor scrapes the embryo from the uterus lining.

Other forms of abortion exist when a pregnancy has gone beyond the twelfth week. Rather than discuss these other procedures, I will just say that a girl should always seek advice from a family-planning organization or a doctor who can counsel her regarding her predicament.

Jan, a college student of mine who got pregnant in high school and had an abortion, told me of her experience. She was very wise, as well as very fortunate, to have had her abortion in a safe, legal manner rather than having a *quickie* abortion at the hands of some incompetent person who would not be particularly concerned about her health and safety: "When I discovered I was pregnant, I didn't know where to turn, so I went to the yellow pages in the phone book and checked for some social service offices. I found the phone number of the Planned Parenthood Clinic and they gave me the phone number for counseling provided by a women's health organization.

"I was given both medical and counseling services for helping me with my pregnancy. I also received a good lecture about why I had not done something to prevent it and how

I could use birth control in the future. Any person can come into the health clinic without being asked about age or marital status. All you need is an appointment for this counseling, although you don't need an appointment for a pregnancy test.

"When I met the counselor I already knew that an abortion was the only answer for me, but I still was not sure deep down that I wanted it. The lady talking to me assured me that an abortion was completely legal since January 22, 1973, when the Supreme Court stated that during the first two trimesters of pregnancy women had a right to make their own decision to have an abortion. They were all very sympathetic toward me and asked me if I would like to see a minister. I don't have one, but I said yes. The lady minister seemed to know all about the guilt and fear I was feeling. She knew the choice was not an easy one to make. It is not like anything else you might decide to do. I may have been putting on a real brave act, but inside I was hurting. She let me know there was no easy answer, but that it was up to me. She could not promise me that I wouldn't have afterthoughts, but she also told me I could come back to her to talk after the abortion was over. She wasn't fooled by my cheerful exterior, and that was good to know.

"After the counselor was convinced that I really preferred an abortion, an appointment was made for me at the abortion clinic. I was given instructions to follow: I was told to be sure to take a bath or shower and to eat a light breakfast of tea and toast before leaving for the clinic. I was not supposed to have anything else but water until after the abortion. I was asked to bring a sanitary belt and a bathrobe. I was advised that I should bring along a friend to drive me home afterwards and not to forget a money order or certified check in the amount of $250 to cover the cost of the abortion.

"The day arrived and I appeared at the clinic with my slip from the clinic attesting that I was no more than twelve weeks pregnant. When I got to the clinic, I had to fill out forms about my past medical history, pay the fee, give a blood and urine sample, see a counselor to talk once more about having an abortion in case I had changed my mind, and then I was put into a little examining room. I was given a robe and told to undress. Then I was brought out into a waiting room with about twenty other women and girls. The wait can be from one to three hours, depending upon how many doctors are there to perform the abortions. While waiting, I had all kinds of feelings. I felt confused, relieved that it would soon be over, frightened over what might go wrong. At times I thought about running out.

"Then I was called into a small room and was told to lie down on a table and put my feet in the stirrups and lift up my gown. The doctor then inserted a tube up my vagina with a needle to freeze my cervix. Then he dilated my cervix by shoving the tube again up into my uterus. Then the nurse turned on the machine, which sucked out the fetus and the extra blood supply. This is done twice to insure getting the fetus. It only takes a few minutes, and it wasn't a very painful process, but it isn't something I'd do again, for I feel I lost part of myself when I had it. I'm going on the Pill before I have sex again. But I am not sorry I had an abortion this time. I could not go to my parents; the guy was not anyone I would want to marry; I knew I was not ready to carry a baby and give birth to it; I knew I could not take care of a baby. I wanted to have a college education, and that is what I am now getting. I feel depressed whenever I think of that abortion, but I know other girls who have had one, and they tell me you get over the depression. And no one except my very closest friends even knows."

If you find yourself in Jan's predicament, you may not choose the alternative of an abortion as she did. None of the choices is easy to make. Guilt seems to prevail regardless of which choice is made. Certainly, the main drawback to having an abortion is the emotional trauma of guilt.

Mary, who had an abortion when she was sixteen, found that her religion helped her through her guilt. "Having an abortion is a scary process, but it couldn't be as bad as what my girlfriend told me she went through when she had her baby," she said. "It did hurt when the doctor put the tube up my vagina with the needle to freeze my cervix, but even that wasn't too bad. But it was such an emotional experience, and a decision that I will have to live with forever. I am a very religious person, and that is what allowed me to cope with the depression and guilt I felt at first. It was a difficult decision, but I knew I would not cause my parents the embarrassment of having a child when not married. They are so highly thought of—just the very best people in our little town."

Most people have very strong feelings about the issue of abortion. Some feel that it is morally wrong; others, that moral considerations do not enter the picture since the fetus is not viable. Whatever the outcome, however, making the decision to have or not have an abortion is a personal one that cannot be made lightly. After the decision is made to have an abortion, it is important that a girl have the support of her boyfriend or a friend or, ideally, her parents. Going through an abortion can be a frightening experience by itself, but to go it alone must be a terribly lonely and fearful thing.

Emily tells about the excellent support she received from the father of her child. She and Chad are a young couple who were deeply in love when she discovered she was pregnant. The timing was wrong, however, and they decided together that an abortion was the best solution for them. Chad's support of Emily helped her through the crisis. She described to me what happened: "The doctor told me I was pregnant. No one knows the helpless feeling of walking out of the doctor's office, tears pouring down my face, not knowing exactly what to do. I knew I should talk with Chad, but I also knew he had to finish college. The only solution would be an abortion.

"When I told Chad he was very shocked, and he was even more upset than I was when I first found out. Poor Chad, it was a couple of days before he got himself back together. Then he became more concerned about my emotional state than about himself. Chad wanted to go right out and get married. But I never even considered it because I loved him too much to want to ruin his chances for his career. He loved me, too, and showed just how much as he supported me in every way in my decision to have an abortion. I set up an appointment to have it on a Friday at the abortion clinic. He paid the cost of $300, and I didn't argue with him because I think it helped him with his guilt—sharing part of the consequences of our love life.

"I was eight weeks pregnant at the time of the abortion. We sat together in the waiting room, anxiously waiting for my call. To be honest, I was scared before I arrived because I didn't know what to expect. But the doctor and nurse talked to us and made me feel very comfortable. Everything went smoothly; very little pain, no tears, only a dizzy feeling from the whole experience. It took about ten minutes, and I walked out with a smile on my face. I was so relieved that everything was over, knowing that there was no baby growing inside me. Chad was relieved also, especially because I took it so well. People always get the impression that an abortion is such a tragic thing. It is not true at all. I guess it really depends on the person. Chad was so concerned about my state of health the following week while we attended our classes at college, it almost made me feel foolish.

"As I write this, it is two years since I had that abortion. Sometimes I think about the baby, and I am so glad I decided the way I did. It was not only fair to Chad and myself, but to the child also. It would not have had much of a chance, for I don't think I could have even loved it. I'm far from being ready for anything like that even now. It would have ruined my chances for my education, and I would not be graduating this June. I know everyone in my family would have been extremely unhappy and embarrassed. Chad and I are no longer lovers. But we still keep in contact, even though he is away in graduate school. Sometimes when he comes home, we even go out on a casual date. He is now engaged to a very lovely graduate student. Again, I am so thankful I had an abortion so that nothing much changed in our lives. Oh, we changed. We grew up a lot, and we will never make love with anyone without taking the necessary precautions to prevent a pregnancy. Why was I so foolish as to think that couldn't happen to me?"

Why not just get married?

The fourth alternative for a pregnant girl is marriage. But unless the couple is ready for the responsibilities of marriage and are in love and intending to get married and have kids right away, this is not one of the better solutions. Statistics for the success of teenage marriages do not paint a very rosy picture. The majority of teenagers who marry do so because of a premarital pregnancy. In fact, about 60 percent of babies born to teenagers are conceived before marriage. Three out of every five such marriages end in divorce within five or six years of marriage.

It is not difficult to understand why these youthful marriages become problem marriages. Usually their limited earning capacity means that many of these young people must live below the level they were probably accustomed to when they lived with their parents. And if they married *only* to give the baby a legitimate name, they will likely feel trapped. The young mother will begin to resent assuming most of the responsibility for caring for a child when she would rather be doing other things that her single friends are doing. The young father will resent having to limit his education and subsequent employment opportunities in order to go out and support his family.

Given the above facts, it does not appear that getting married for the sake of giving a child legitimacy is a good idea. Of course, if the young couple receives support from their parents—living with them, for instance, or getting financial support to finish their education and the like—then they may get along better.

The following is an account of five teenage couples in the age bracket of seventeen to nineteen who got married because of a premarital pregnancy. Of course, their names are fictitious.

Sheila and Burt were married at the age of seventeen, and their daughter was born six months later. They are living with his parents, who have a much lower income than Sheila's parents. She is not happy, and they both consider themselves trapped. "We have one small bedroom to call our own. We have absolutely no privacy and his mother is always prying into our business. Just because we are living with them, she thinks she should know everything about us. They are a back-stabbing family and are always making comments about my folks. My parents did not want me to get married, so they won't support us now. Mom wanted me to go to Wyoming to visit an aunt and, then after the baby was born, to give it up for adoption. Dad said I should have an abortion to save everyone disgrace. My friends thought my pregnancy was great but after I went back to finish my last semester, they turned away from me. Burt's mother insisted he had to marry me, but his dad and also his priest suggested he join the Marines. Now his dad is not happy about the extra expense, but his mom says they have to help us out.

"At first I felt very cheated, but now I feel that way only when I think that my folks would have paid my way through college," Sheila concluded.

Burt added, "I didn't plan to go to college, but I sure won't be able to do a lot of the things I did want to do. I still go out a lot more than Sheila. If she can't find a baby-sitter, she can't go out. She also has to make her plans two or three weeks ahead of time. Having a baby isn't nearly as great as we thought it would be. Actually, we never tried not to have one, and she even said she would like to get pregnant. Maybe she thought it would be cool to really get her mom upset. She sure did, and now we are both sorry."

Mary and Dick were eighteen when they were married, and their daughter was born four months later. Both their families were in the upper-income bracket. The couple is living with Mary's parents, and they are very appreciative of their parents' help. She told me, "I don't know where we would be now if it weren't for them." Dick added, "Mary doesn't know how to cook and she has never taken care of a baby before. Her mom has taken over our daughter's care. Her parents are great, and we are both able to finish our college education."

When I asked Mary and Dick what their parents' reactions were to the news that she was pregnant, she said, "Nobody told me what I had to do. Mother was enthused about becoming a grandmother. Dad thought I should either get married or have an abortion. I felt pressured within myself because I wasn't sure Dick would want to get married now, although we loved each other very much and were planning to get married when we finished college. When we were married, none of the relatives and only a few close friends even knew I was pregnant. Dick's parents were rather distant, and his mom acted as though I was taking her boy away from her."

Dick added, "I was really surprised that there were no pressures. My folks said it was up to me; although Mom hinted about an abortion, she never came right out and said so. My sister went through the same situation and things worked out great for her, so I am not too worried so long as the parents continue to help us."

Mary went on, "As wonderful as the folks are with the baby, I still can't go out as often as I would like. I feel I should stay home and play the mother role, but my mother keeps telling me she will take care of the baby. I used to do a lot of silk-screening, and now Daddy wants me to get back into this. I might, but right now I have lost my enthusiasm." Dick added that he has less time to do things he wants to do, but he is not complaining. "We certainly didn't deliberately try to have a baby. Mary's doctor had told her she was very underdeveloped inside, so she thought this meant she couldn't get pregnant. But instead she gave birth to a very healthy, eight-pound baby. And now we are married as planned, but four years ahead of schedule."

Jean and Paul were both eighteen when they were married, and their baby girl was born eight months later. They have their own apartment, filled with hand-me-downs. Paul went right to work in a factory, as he had planned to do when he finished high school. When Jean became pregnant, her parents insisted she should get married right away. "They also told me if I did not want to get married, I could go away and visit relatives until after the baby was born and it was given away for adoption. But since Paul and I had planned on getting married in a few months anyway, hurrying it up didn't upset things too much," added Jean. Paul's parents weren't so anxious for him to marry. He told me, "They put the pressure on for me to encourage Jean to give the baby up for adoption. My brothers thought I was crazy to get married. Jean's mom was more concerned about what the neighbors would say than anything."

When asked if she ever regrets getting married so young, Jean answered, "I'm not able to do all the things I could if I weren't married, and if we didn't have our baby. But I enjoy doing things with Paul. The responsibilities of caring for our baby hold me down, and sometimes I feel as if I am being denied the chance to explore. Sometimes I think I don't have any talents, and now I won't have much opportunity to find out. Paul wants me to take up guitar lessons, and when our baby gets older, maybe I will." Paul said, "I am perfectly happy with the way things are. Having a baby made us grow up fast, and we have become better friends to each other. Of course, we feel sorry for ourselves when we can't even afford a can of beer right before payday. My parents can't afford to help us, and Jean's parents have got four other younger children at home. We didn't intend for Jean to get pregnant before we were married, but I think it is great. She is such a beautiful baby—I hope we won't have any more kids, though, for a long time, because we have so many bills."

Betty and Bill also were eighteen when they were married, and their baby was born six months later. They, too, have their own apartment. They are very poor, but so were their own parents. Betty told me, "My parents were furious and ashamed of me when I told them I was pregnant. They suggested an abortion. But when I wouldn't go for that, they said we should get married. Bill's parents didn't say anything. Neither Bill nor I planned on going to college, but I wanted to go on to a trade school. We surely didn't want to have a baby, but I don't know why we didn't do something to prevent it. I always watched the calendar for when I couldn't become pregnant. One night when we were making love, I can remember thinking how nice it would be to have a baby with him, and I bet that was the night it happened. Bill would always ask me if it was a safe time and, at first, he was mad that I fooled him. But then he accepted it.

"Now that I have a baby to take care of I realize that I have cheated myself out of any independence. It would be nice to have a job of my own, maybe my own place with some money to spend on clothes. Instead we have to scrimp, scrimp, just like our folks. These feelings build up inside of me and then I realize how selfish I am being. Bill is selfish sometimes, too, because we can't afford a baby-sitter and he thinks he can go out without me. My mother has a way of reminding me that we asked for this when we got ourselves a baby, so I don't ask her to baby-sit very often. What worries me is that we fight a lot, and sometimes we really go too far and take a sock at each other."

Bill said, "We are really too young for the responsibility of having a kid and, financially, we would have been better off if we could have waited for a couple of years. Who knows, by then we might not have even gotten married."

These four marriages are all less than a year old. Certainly it is too early to make any predictions about their outcomes. Mary and Dick, whose parents are in the upper-income bracket and willing to support them while they both complete their college education, seem to be quite happy with their marriage and having a baby. Jean and Paul were very much in love and had planned to marry in the near future. They are satisfied with their marriage and have a realistic view of themselves and their future. The parents of both these couples are supportive of them.

Sheila and Burt, who were only seventeen when they became parents, have been forced to live with his parents. They both say they are sorry about the whole situation. In addition, Sheila resents the fact that she has lost her opportunity to have her parents put her through college. Betty and

Bill are living in poverty with little or no emotional support
from their parents. They both feel trapped. They would not
have married if she had not become pregnant. Neither of
these two couples receives financial or much emotional support from their parents.

While a majority of marriages that take place because of
a premarital pregnancy do end in divorce or separation, many
are successful. Bev and Ron have had a satisfying marriage for
fifteen years, though she finds that she still feels guilty about
her premarital pregnancy:

"It just happened. And only once. That night in April—
but getting pregnant was an impossibility in our minds. I was
almost eighteen, and he was nineteen, a freshman in college.
My period was late for the first time in my life. I suspected
my plight, and in my shame I broke off with my boyfriend. I
didn't want it to happen again, and I never even told him why
I wouldn't see him. He kept calling me. When I graduated from
high school, I got a full-time job. I was a big girl so my condition remained hidden for a long time. My mother didn't notice my morning sickness—she was always too busy to pay me
any attention. I think Dad suspected, but he never said a word.
Ron kept calling. September arrived and I announced that I
wasn't going to college—wanted to continue with my job.

"Then one night he came over and insisted that we talk.
I confessed my situation, and he told me he loved me and
talked me into getting married. We had blood tests, and only
on the day that we went for our license did I tell my parents
we were getting married—but not about my pregnancy. My
mother wouldn't speak to me. She was furious that I chose
marriage over going to college. He had told his parents the
whole story, and although they were upset, they accepted the
idea. My parents wouldn't attend our wedding and closed
their eyes to us for a time. The last thing my mother said to
me before I left the house for my wedding was, 'Well, at least
I hope you'll use birth control.' And I said, 'Sorry Mom, it's
too late for that now.' His parents came to our wedding and
had a cake afterwards at their house. Then we went to our
newly rented furnished apartment. A couple of months later
Mom and Dad came over to our apartment to see. She never

said she was sorry about her actions at our wedding, but I think she was. Dad was just his old self. At least we were friends again with my parents.

"We had been married just seven weeks when our son was born. We loved each other, and we loved our baby. Financially, things were tough, and we were not happy that he had to leave college to take a job in a factory. We were not going to ask for help—and I don't know if we would have received it anyhow. We were determined to solve our own problems. Then it became necessary for me to find a job. He was working the second shift and could be home with the baby while I worked during the day. I found a well-paying office job, and we found a nice grandmother-type baby-sitter when he decided to get a second job. It was our plan to get ahead, and then for him to return to college.

"He did finally graduate from college. We have had a good marriage, but my sexual adjustment has not been the best. For me, sex just isn't important. But if he is satisfied, so am I. I am sure this is because I still feel guilty about my premarital pregnancy. He can't understand how I can still feel guilty, but it's more than that. It's not my past but my children's future I worry about. Will I blame my son at some time for not being able to have the career I wanted? Do I take it out on him when I'm angry? I have always been harder on my oldest son than on my other two children. My main worry is what he will think of me if he learns he was conceived before our marriage. How can we teach values and morality if we, ourselves, have put ours aside for a moment? Will the years of his childhood, in which we have tried to be honest with him, cancel our past mistake? I wish I could find answers to these questions."

These five examples of marriage that took place because of a premarital pregnancy give some idea of the problems that can occur. Most studies of school-age marriages show that chances for unhappiness, separation, and divorce are far, far greater than chances for happiness and a lasting marriage.

So when you ask me which is the *best* alternative for a pregnant girl, I have to say each alternative has its own problems. The choice depends on your individual situation. None is without pain.

When a girl is only sixteen or seventeen, does her age affect the chances of having a healthy baby?

According to studies done by Gabriel Stickle and supported by the National Foundation/March of Dimes in New York City in 1974 and 1975, the infant mortality rate for babies born to mothers under fifteen is about 44 per 1000 infants, compared to 31 per 1000 for mothers between the ages of fifteen and nineteen and 22 per thousand for mothers between the ages of twenty and twenty-four.[5] The younger the mother, the smaller the chances of survival for the infant.

A study made by W. C. Opel in 1971 shows that babies born to mothers under eighteen are more likely to be underweight at birth, more likely to grow up having behavioral problems and a lower IQ.[6] These conditions may also exist because many teenage mothers have inadequate diets and suffer from malnutrition. They are living at poverty level or are living with parents at poverty level, so they don't get proper medical care and can't afford some of the advantages that contribute to healthy and intelligent children. Most of these young people lack education themselves, and their inability to rear an infant patiently into adulthood is directly related to the difficulties mentioned.

I've heard that teenage parents often are child abusers. Is this true?

Recent reports indicate that teenage parents are very likely to become child abusers.[7] Child abusers who neglect their children, as Marge did in leaving her baby unattended, or who physically and emotionally harm their children, are usually people under pressure. Child abuse occurs among both the rich and the poor, but the percentage is higher among the poor. The teenage mother living on welfare does not have money for baby-sitters when she wants to go out and have

fun with her friends. It is frustrating not being able to have
the comforts that perhaps she was used to having while living
at home with her parents. She may feel resentful of her child,
blaming it for her plight. Normal childhood behavior such as
refusing to finish a meal, crying, waking up before it is time,
wetting a diaper, become excuses for verbal or physical
attacks.

For example, a teenager may interpret crying as a symbol
of rejection. One teenage mother said to me, "When my baby
cries, I feel as though she doesn't love me." If this young
girl has been rejected by her parents, she may be particularly
sensitive to feeling rejected by her child. She then may slap
out at her child with violence.

Many teenagers have unrealistic expectations about a
child's physical and mental development. They have been
known to punish a baby for not sitting up alone at the age
of twelve weeks, when a child is not physically developed for
this until it is about twenty-seven or twenty-eight weeks old!

Various forms of child abuse include bruising and beat-
ing, burning with cigarettes, stoves, hot water and other
liquids, and with electrical appliances such as irons and
toasters (I have seen a picture of a five-month-old child who
had deep burns on her behind from being set on a steam ra-
diator to dry her diaper); human bites, missing teeth, stab
wounds, gouged-out eyes, and sexual abuse; physical neglect,
such as not giving a child proper food, clothing, and medical
care; emotional neglect, when a parent blames the child for
its predicament and does not seem to care for the child; and
verbal abuse. A good example of verbal abuse is when a
mother says to her child, "If it weren't for you, I wouldn't
be in this mess. You are just like your father, he is as rotten
as they come." A child brought up hearing such talk can
very well develop a low sense of self-esteem.

Can anything be done about child abuse? Just recently I
saw a young mother yanking a six- or seven-month-old child
around by the arm and finally slapping it in the face when he
cried. I couldn't stand by and see this without asking this
young girl if she didn't realize how much she was hurting her

little baby. Somewhat surprised at my interference, she said, "Oh, I know it, but I get so I just can't stand this kid. He cries all the time anyway." DeLissovoy reports seeing many babies being hit in the face or spanked brutally by their adolescent mother or father.

Reports of child abuse continue, and until teenage mothers can be discouraged from keeping their babies when they are in no social, financial, or emotional state to care for themselves or their child, we will see a continued rise of child abuse among teenage parents. This situation can be helped through educational programs for teenage parents so that they will better understand the problems and responsibilities that go with having a baby. They need to realize the tremendous changes and adjustments that will take place in their lives and in relationships with their families and friends. Such programs can teach teenage parents child care and what they can expect from their baby as it grows and develops. Young people need help, too, in realizing the importance of sacrificing some of their independence in order to be able to complete their education and make plans for a career: Living with parents can be difficult, but it may be the best idea for the baby's well-being, if not for the teenage mother.

Maturity usually increases with age, and the teenager generally has a distance to go before she develops enough of it to give patient, tender, loving care to a child. Of course, not all young parents are potential child abusers. Many of them have a sense of maturity beyond their age. They want their babies, and they are loving and tender with them. It is true that all parents, at some time or other, are impatient with or abusive to their children. But it is also true that school-age parents present the greatest likelihood for becoming child abusers, just by the nature of their situation.

How does having a baby affect a single girl's chances for dating and her social life in general?

According to a study by F. Ivan Nye, the girl who becomes pregnant in her teens has few life choices left for her to make. Ninety percent of her choices are already made when she finds she is pregnant. That is, her chance of completing her education is limited, her choice of a mate may be far less (and is nil if she marries her baby's father because of her pregnancy), her relationship with her friends becomes difficult or at least different, so that many pregnant girls feel slighted or rejected by their social groups. Certainly with a baby to look after, her freedom to come and go as she pleases seldom continues.[8]

A baby cannot be taken on dates, and few school-age mothers can support a baby-sitter. Grandmothers may help, and most of them do. But responsibility for the child is really up to its mother. She probably will have to drop out of school. Only 17.5 percent of girls between the ages of sixteen and seventeen who have babies graduate from high school, and only 39 percent of girls between the ages of eighteen and nineteen.[9] Lacking an education, a teenage mother will have trouble finding a job that pays enough for her to live alone and support her baby. That welfare check does not go very far, either. Thus, she may be forced to live at home, or to marry someone she doesn't really want to marry. She will be subjected to her parents' disapproval of her actions. She will be subjected to snubs by a society that still looks down on a girl who has a baby out of wedlock. Men may think she is an "easy lay," and they may not even want to consider marrying a young woman with a child.

What about the father of the baby? Doesn't he have any responsibility for what happens?

Unfortunately, it seems that society tends to forget that a pregnancy requires sperm as well as an ovum! The girl gets the attention, criticism, responsibility when she becomes pregnant. The woman alone must carry the baby for nine months, serving as a reminder of what *she* has done. So she must carry the emotional brunt as well. Arguments are heard pro and con about whether a man should have a voice in what the girl does about her pregnancy. In asking my students about this sticky issue I found that the men and women were equally unsure of what they would do in such a situation.

Jane said, "If the couple was going steady and having sex because they loved each other, then I think they should make a joint decision as to what *they* will do about a pregnancy. But if a teenage boy and girl were having sex just for the hell of it, with no commitment, then I think the girl will find the boy really has no interest in what she would decide to do about a pregnancy. Furthermore, I don't think he would have any right to tell her what to do."

Lynn wanted to give her baby up for adoption and she tells what happened to her: "Bill and I were just casual friends who enjoyed sex now and then. When I first told him I was pregnant, he called me stupid for letting it happen. He stayed clear of me after that. Well, I had the baby, and since I was only seventeen, I agreed with my folks that I should give the baby up for adoption. To our surprise, our state requires that you name the father in court and have your name published once in some newspaper, giving notice to the father to come forth and sign the release papers.

"I did this and that guy came to court and refused to sign the release. Here I am at nineteen with a three-year-old son, unmarried, and my parents have the care of my baby on their hands. Bill gives me money for child support, but he's leaving the state soon, and who knows what he will do about payments then."

Most of the fellows agreed that the father of a child should have some rights to decide what will happen to their baby. They also felt that these fathers should uphold their responsibilities and give the mother of their child emotional and financial support after the decision is reached.

John very strongly felt that if he got a girl pregnant, he would want her to decide what she wanted to do, since it was her body and she would be much more affected by going through a pregnancy than he.

Tom felt the decision should be up to both. As he said: "A girl doesn't get into that situation by herself. The guy must share responsibility, and they must have a very serious discussion about various ways of handling this. If marriage is out of the question, then how about having the baby and giving it up for adoption? If abortion becomes the only realistic solution, then go with her to a clinic and help her all the way with your support, for the experience and the decision belongs to you *both*."

Many young men, according to Ivan Nye's study, accept their responsibility and try to fulfill it. Forty percent of young men marry the girl who carries their child. And almost two-thirds of young unwed fathers contribute financial help, at least for a while.[10] Many young men have guilt feelings about the premarital pregnancy and often regret what has happened as much as the girl. A very few men consider that getting a girl pregnant and not helping her is something to brag about.

It appears that although it is the girl who is "stuck" with the consequences of sex without responsible birth control, the majority of unwed fathers help out to some degree.

A premarital pregnancy has negative consequences for the father, too. If he marries the girl, that early marriage is very likely to interrupt his education and he is more likely to remain in unskilled, lower-paying jobs for the rest of his life. He also has a high chance of a divorce.

As we have said earlier, the father of a child born out of wedlock does have a legal responsibility, regardless of his age or whether he marries the mother, provided it is proven he is the father or he voluntarily accepts responsibility. He can be sued for child support until the child reaches legal age. He can be sued, fined, and imprisoned for committing statutory rape (intercourse with a girl under *the age of consent*), which is a felony charge in most states, even though the girl may have given her consent. In addition, men have feelings, too, and can suffer pangs of guilt and fear and go through emotional traumas similar to what girls may go through when it is learned that there is a pregnancy and choices must be made.

A young man who objects to an abortion hurts emotionally when a girl aborts his child. When a girl keeps a child,

he hurts financially, too. When she gives their child up for
adoption, he must wonder about what happened to his child,
just as she wonders. If he feels obligated to marry the girl,
even though he does not love her or want even to think of
getting married, he has many other emotional and social burdens to carry.

*Why should my mother and father be so upset over my preg-
nancy? After all, I am the one having the baby.*

Parents usually consider what their children do as a reflection
of themselves. When you become pregnant, they can not help
but wonder what they did wrong in bringing you up. Parents
probably suffer more pain when something unfortunate happens to their child than the child feels.

Families of unmarried pregnant girls worry about their
daughters, but even more, they worry about their prospective
grandchild. They generally are aware of the hardships that
can lie ahead for their daughters as well as for their grandchildren. In addition, many are worried about social disgrace
and added financial burdens.

Your parents are legally responsible for you until you
are eighteen. And now they will have the additional care
of a baby.

The most usual immediate response of parents to the
news of a premarital pregnancy is shock, then anger, and then
sorrow for their daughter, whose happy, carefree days are
gone forever. While most mothers look forward to the day
they become grandmothers, this is far from what they
planned. Chances are it is your mother who will end up
helping you care for your child. It doesn't matter that she
may want some freedom from household and child-rearing
chores, now that you and your siblings are grown up. How
can she be happy about being tied down now with the responsibilities of caring for a grandchild, no matter how much
she may love that child? If you and she want you to continue
your education, she is going to be tied down for several more
years.

Then think of your father. He is concerned about your mother's added responsibility. He feels that you should be the one to stay home and care for your baby, whereas you want to get out more with your friends. Can you blame him for not being happy about the added cost of providing for your baby at the time he thought he would be able to begin saving for his retirement? Your parents are disappointed, for they had hoped that when they did become grandparents, you would be married to a man you loved who would be able to provide well for you and your child.

As we have seen, in the past few years more and more babies are being born to single school-age parents. Not only the girl, but the boy, his parents, and her parents, all the other members of the family, and all of society to a certain extent, are involved in a premarital pregnancy. Regardless of which decision is made—marriage, abortion, single parenthood, adoption—everyone is hurt to a varying degree. Prevention of pregnancy through an effective means of contraception clearly is the ideal solution. Another solution is recognition that you do have choices available. That is, you can decide not to have sexual intercourse until you are married. This is still a popular choice, and most fellows are willing to go along with their girl's choice to be married as a virgin.

7 living together versus getting married

IN THE LAST three or four years, more and more high-school students have asked me questions about the advantages of living together over marriage. They are reflecting the increased openness in our society about men and women living together without benefit of a marriage certificate. About two million unrelated and unmarried women and men are sharing living quarters, according to the Population Reference Bureau. The largest increase in living together is found within younger age groups, particularly college students and young adults starting out in new jobs in cities away from their families. Over one-third of these young unmarried couples live together a relatively short time (about four and a half months) before they either marry or separate.[1]

Why are we finding an increase in living together without the benefit of marriage among young people?

We do not find many high-school students living together, for obvious reasons. They are usually living with their parents and do not have the necessary income to set up a living-together arrangement. College students living away from home, on the other hand, may see living together as a substitute for being at home. As Larry said, "I was alone on a big campus and lonesome as hell separated from my family and my old friends. When Liza moved in with me, it gave me the sense of *family*—and besides, it was much cheaper sharing the rent and other household expenses. She did the shopping and cooking and I did the housework and laundry. We loved each other as good friends. But, we weren't interested in each

other sexually, since we both had *steadies* at home, so we
slept in twin beds. Needless to say, we didn't tell our steadies
or our parents. But we weren't doing anything wrong, and
besides, it's considered the okay thing to do on campus. At
the end of the semester, we agreed to split. Guess our con-
sciences got to us."

Our society is becoming more accepting of new and different kinds of behavior and so more people are feeling freer
to "do their own thing" even if only for a short period of
time. When you are living on a large campus where you are
just a little cog in a huge wheel, you can't help but feel a
sense of separateness. You also will experience a sense of
privacy in being away from everyone you know back home,
which allows you the feeling of freedom to behave in ways
you wouldn't have living at home.

In addition to the need for feelings of being close to
someone, the desire for sex, and economic reasons, some
people are living together instead of marrying because they
are afraid of marriage. Recent reports indicate that the young
people most in favor of living together without marriage are
those who had unloving, negative relationships with their
parents. Failing to see marriage as a way to achieve the close
relationships that most everyone seems to need and desire,
they reject marriage and turn to other life-styles.[2]

How does living together happen and what is it like?

Living together has different meanings for different people,
depending on their situation and needs or expectations.
Some students explained their relationships as something
that just happened as their dating became more serious.
Jackie, for example, told me, "One night we decided he
should stay over with me and after that he stayed more and
more nights and weekends, until finally he just moved in with
me."

Various studies of cohabitation show that deciding to
live together is often this kind of gradual drifting into
staying together. This arrangement usually involves sleeping

together, for most couples are already deeply involved
sexually. However, there are some men and women living
together in sort of a "buddy" relationship like Larry's living
arrangement with Liza.

Living together is actually like being married in many
ways. There is some commitment to each other. The couple
establishes a household. Rent must be paid, furniture ac-
quired, decisions made on who does which chores. Adjustments must be made to each other's habits. And dissolving
a living-together relationship has problems similar to a
divorce, as will be discussed later.

*Doesn't living together rather than getting married actually
make more sense? Isn't it better to find out about each other
in this way before you get married?*

Many students think that living together is a good way to
learn how to get along with another person, and to obtain
greater knowledge of what living with another person involves. It is important to have this kind of information, of
course, and living with a roommate can teach something
about accommodating one's needs and values to those of
another and compromising. Advantages in living together
without benefit of marriage, then, are: ready sex without
strings, freedom to walk out at any time, sharing the costs
and work involved in keeping a household, and companionship.

But there are obvious disadvantages too, and some that
are not so obvious—lack of emotional commitment, underlying guilt, fear of being found out, the family's disapproval
and scorn, missing out on other possible dates, finding a
satisfactory place to rent where a couple can live together unmarried, the fact that any resultant children would be considered illegitimate, and various legal problems, such as
community property laws and rights of inheritance.

I find it interesting that in the discussions I've had with
college students about this very subject, more men than
women seem to have doubts about the benefits of living to-

gether. For instance, Tom discusses what he considers a major disadvantage of living together—lack of emotional commitment. As he said: "If a guy and a girl want to live together before marriage to see how it is, I would expect that they are very unsure of themselves and want an easy way out if things don't work out. To me, living together indicates that the relationship is not strong enough to warrant marriage or that one is using the other to satisfy his personal sex need. He has his money and the *no-strings-attached sex*—'Oh, so you are pregnant, bye!' The girl has no legal way to get back at him, and she is left holding the bag, so to speak. If a gal wants to live with him, what has *he* got to lose? Maybe a broken heart if she decides to leave him and he really loves her."

Bill added, "You can live together without a firm commitment being made. That allows you to part if this togetherness does not realize your expectations. But it's just so easy you may tend *not* to work at staying together if a problem should appear. If you want a longer, more binding commitment, then marry."

Nineteen-year-old Clarence was emphatic as he exclaimed, "I'm not in favor of two people living together without a commitment. And believe me, the commitment makes the difference. I've seen couples who have lived together for two or three years and were fighting half the time, but as soon as they had the paper signed, the change started, because they had something real to cling to—a legal commitment."

Because of the lack of emotional commitment, many living-together arrangements are unstable and last for only short periods of time. Some individuals find it very miserable changing from one partner to another. Janet tells how frustrated she became, always hoping the next relationship would be happy and lasting: "I lived with Jerry my third semester after going with him for a couple of months. He left after two months when he decided he had enough of 'putting up with me,' as he said. I was so lonely that I began to negotiate right away with Mike, hoping he would like me better. He quit college at the end of the semester and I was devastated because I really liked Mike. He left without even feeling sorry about ending our relationship. There must really be something wrong with me because the longest any guy has ever stayed with me is about four months. Now at the end of my sophomore year, I've lived with three guys and they all have left. My last roommate, Rob, has transferred to another college. I think I've learned something. Without an emotional commitment, a relationship isn't going to work or last. These guys enjoyed sex with me and they liked my cooking, but they weren't very unhappy at all when they left. I've been miserable, and I think I'll find some girls to live with after this."

Jill presents another popular view of the importance of commitment, which is lacking in living together: "By dating long enough, you should be aware of each other's faults and good points. Living together isn't the right thing to do. If the courtship is long enough and is gone into the right way, there should be no apprehension about getting married. Besides, being married is never the same as living together. Living together can put a strain on a relationship if the two are not prepared for the pitfalls, just as in a marriage. This may be useful for some couples, and many couples who live together eventually end up getting married. But I think if we advocated this rather than marriage, we would end up with a lot of confused and hurt people walking around, not to mention unwanted and unplanned-for children."

Underlying guilt, as stated earlier, is a significant disadvantage to living together. Guilt feelings exist when a girl has been reared in a family or in a religious faith that taught her that she should marry before she lives with a man. It is always difficult to behave in ways that we know are disapproved by those we love and respect, even if we ourselves believe that what we are doing is right.

Mary talked about underlying guilt feelings and the possible family strain that can occur when you live with a person outside of marriage: "My cousin lived with a guy for two years, and my mother and dad were very accepting about it, although her parents were very upset by it. When she and her boyfriend came to visit us, we were all prepared for them to share a room as if they were married. But when bedtime came, she just *flipped out* and began to cry so hard that they left and did not come back. I heard her tell my mother she just could not do this in a house with young kids. A year later, after they were married, she told me that even their sex life was different and better, knowing that everyone approved."

Betty told about her experience of living with her boyfriend Ron. "I was working, and he was attending college, and it just seemed the thing to do, so we moved in together. It was very cozy, and we spent a lot of time together. He had lots more free time than I, so to my surprise he did most of the cooking and housecleaning. It seemed just as if we were playing house. We frequently engaged in sexual intercourse, but I was always worrying so much about getting pregnant and about what my mother would think if she knew we were living together, that I never really was satisfied. After about a year, I began to feel different about things. We weren't talking or doing things together like before. My feelings were changing for him. He seemed more like a brother to me than a lover. I don't know why, but that's what happened.

"We began to realize that we had rushed into living together too fast, and we were not at all ready for anything as mature as marriage. We had to pay for the consequences in many ways. It was really sad to see Ron's face. He looked so sad and sober and very empty and lonely, because he still wanted me. Now that I'm older, I have a much more serious attitude toward sex and love and marriage. It takes a lot of responsibility and a mature attitude to handle it in the right way."

Gary said, "I have been dating a girl for over a year, and we have gotten to know each other in all the important ways just as well as living together. The only things we don't know about each other are how we brush our teeth and what soap we prefer for a shower and little stuff like that. And who really cares about such details? I know my parents would have been so embarrassed if we had moved in together, and they don't have to know that we have been having sexual intercourse. They can guess about it, but they don't have to know for sure and neither does anyone else."

John thinks parents will get over their bitterness about their kids living together if the kids get married or after they break up the relationship. "My mom thought it was terrible to move in with my girlfriend right after I graduated from high school. But she had a job, and it seemed like the thing to do. Mom asked me to keep it quiet from the rest of the family. Now that I am no longer living with this girl, Mom thinks I am okay again."

While John's mother knew about his relationship, and Mary's parents accepted but disapproved of her cousin's relationship, Betty expressed the *fear of being found out.* This fear is felt by most college students unless they have parents who they know can be accepting of their living together. When a couple is trying to hide their relationship from friends and family, they are denying themselves the support these people could give in times of stress. Liz and David went to their parents and told them they were going to live together until he finished graduate school. They expressed their commitment to each other and their intent to get married after graduation and both sets of parents accepted their decision. Liz was nineteen, David twenty-two, and their parents continued to give both emotional and financial support as before. After two years this couple is very satisfied with their life-style.

Obviously, their parents did not have the sexual hang-ups that many have. They probably speculated that their kids were sexually involved, but they didn't ask or demand a definite answer. I think this is the greatest cause of family strain over a young person's living with someone of the opposite sex. The first thing that comes to mind is *sex*, and since this has been given such a dirty connotation, parents are very embarrassed when they find out and are forced to admit that their children are living together outside of marriage. Unmarried cohabitation, of course, is contrary to all of our religious and social rules, regulations, customs, and values.

Ruthie tells of other problems she and her steady had when they decided to live together. "We didn't realize how difficult just finding a place was going to be. We finally found a landlord who didn't care that we weren't married—just so we paid the rent. But then whose name should we put on the mailbox, since we didn't want the neighbors to know we weren't married? We finally put a hyphenated name on the mailbox—his last name and mine. But if we thought this was a problem, it was nothing compared to the worry I had about getting pregnant. After a year, we got a little careless and I did get pregnant. He was angry and threatened to leave unless I got an abortion. That was entirely against my religion and I wouldn't, so he did walk out on me, telling me I was so stupid, getting pregnant. I don't really know how I will handle an illegitimate child at this moment. I do wish I had never met its father, or lived with him."

It seems the above commentaries have stressed the disadvantages more than the advantages. However, college girls generally seem to see more positive rationales for living together before marriage than do the fellows. Marge expressed a majority view by saying, "If you live with someone rather than getting married, you don't have the legal ties of a license or a commitment to the other person. I think it is great to learn about the opposite sex and find out his way of doing things before marriage because if you were married and divorce came about, there would be too many legal ties that have to be broken. You can get firsthand experience in what spending your life with someone will be like before you tie the knot. I don't feel you ever really know someone well enough to pledge your life to him until you live with him."

Granted, there are advantages to living together, for one can learn many things about the habits and attitudes of a person before tying the knot. Having regular sexual experience if and when you want it can be great, and if things don't turn out you can split without the expense of a divorce.

Eileen had a very positive living-together experience. She explained: "We were going steady in high school and when

we went away to college, we decided to live together. Our
folks were disappointed and embarrassed, but actually I don't
think they were too surprised at our wanting to be together.
They don't say much, and when we go home for visits, we
each sleep in our own homes. We are both working our way
through college, and this way's much cheaper. We had sex
before this, but now it is much more satisfying not to have
to find a safe place or to rush. We really get to know each
other's way of doing things, our likes and dislikes. When we
get angry or upset, we talk it out, which is the way our
parents do. While we know we could split without a divorce,
we have too strong a commitment to do that very easily. We
agreed that if by the time we finish college either one of us
didn't want to continue our relationship, we would break up.
After two years, we are now making plans ahead for our marriage with a great deal of assurance that we really are right
for each other."

Eileen's living-together arrangement is not typical of cohabitation among college students. As shown earlier, most
young people who live together do not marry. More likely,
by living together, you will risk the feelings of guilt over
doing things your parents disapprove of, as well as fear that
your parents will catch on. You may suffer tension over
your awareness that you can walk out on each other at any
time, and risk the probable emotional hurt when your partnership breaks up. In addition, you miss out on other dates
that might lead to marriage.

*My friend wants to live with a guy, and I don't think she's
ready. How can I convince her she is making a mistake?*

I would talk to your friend, giving her information such as
that discussed above so that she understands both the advantages and disadvantages of living together before making her
choice. As Alan advises: "I think you should talk to your
friend about her plans. Try to help her see it from all angles.
In the process, you will get a chance to express yourself.
Remember, everyone chooses his own course in life, and you

can be responsible for only yourself. You can talk together so she can examine her choice, but there is no use in placing pressure on her to change her mind. I assume she feels alienated from her parents, fearing they would object, so be cautious in how you express yourself, to keep your lines of communication open to her. She needs someone to talk to. She will make her own decisions; you must accept that."

"Ask your friend to look hard and objectively at her reasons for wanting to live with a man," suggests Marie. "Ask her to tell you if she really believes it is morally right for her. Ask her to weigh the facts carefully and see *why* it's so important to her. Then ask what objections she has to marriage. What about him? Why do they fear it? If you have made her think objectively and realistically and if she has looked into her long-range goals (what kind of future she has with this man, what about his education, his values?), I think you have done the best you can to help her. The decision is hers."

When you live together, what about seeing other people?

As I said earlier, living together is most often an outgrowth of going steady together. Usually this means you've given up any intention of going with others. On the other hand, if the relationship is just a matter of convenience between friends, and both decide that each has the right to date others, then, of course, seeing others would be okay. If you *can* date others while living together, you won't be subject to the disadvantage of losing opportunities to meet other people who might be much more suitable for marriage.

What happens when two people split up after living together? Isn't it a lot easier than getting a divorce?

Dissolving a living-together arrangement may not involve the cost of a divorce, but there are likely to be legal entanglements to resolve. For example, in most states, marriage gives the wife some ownership of her husband's property, such as their home and furnishings. When a girl and a fellow live together outside marriage, there is no joint ownership. Whoever bought the furniture owns it. Thus, there can be a hassle proving who bought what and deciding who gets what.

Children are illegitimate and if the child is left with the mother, many legal problems may ensue in order to obtain financial support from the father if he does not volunteer it. The illegitimate child, in most states, has no claim on his father's estate in case of his father's death unless the father included the child in his will. Similarly, in most states, the man and the woman who live together have no claim on each other's estates in case of their deaths unless they have written wills.

Emotional problems are part of a living-together relationship, in many ways similar to those in a marriage. When a couple decides to live together there are usually supportive, affectionate feelings existing between the two. When they separate, it is very possible for the one who may still be in love to feel real grief over the loss of this once-intimate relationship. A deliberate rejection is very difficult to accept without feeling hurt. Even the one who wanted out will feel a sense of change that can be very disturbing. Learning to live alone again can be a very lonely task, and persons who have lived together and then separate can feel the same sense of depression as a person who has been divorced. This may be the reason that so many young people very quickly get involved in another living-together arrangement after the breakup of their previous relationship.

Living together, therefore, is very much like marriage, with many of the same problems, and dissolving such a relationship has many similarities to getting a divorce.

What can I do to help my parents get over their bitterness toward me for going against their wishes and living with a guy? Now that we are getting married, do you think my mom and dad should pay for my wedding?

This depends on the individual situation. Most parents look forward to the marriage of their children. When a son or daughter chooses to live with someone without marriage, it is a disappointment. Some parents accept the choice as being up to their child. Others find acceptance impossible. Whenever we do anything contrary to what our parents or society thinks is right, we must be willing to pay the penalties. Having a bitter parent or one who refuses to pay for a wedding may be the penalty you have to pay for making your choice to live with a man without that *piece of paper.*

Mrs. Brown, an older college student and a mother of three, was adamant in her reaction to this situation: "How can anyone expect her parents to pay for the wedding or to forget how badly she made them feel? My daughter did this to me and my husband, and though I have forgiven her, I shall not forget all the embarrassment she caused us and the rest of the kids. I hope they will decide to get married, but when they do, it should be just a small wedding. How could she even think of having a regular wedding with white dress and veil after what she has done?"

In many cases this bitterness does go away as the wedding date approaches, however. As Julie said, "My parents were so happy when I told them we were getting married that they forgave us for living together and are giving us a big wedding."

Kathy, too, has a happy story to tell. "My folks were very disappointed in me for living with my boyfriend, even though he was four years older and had a job. After my mother saw that we really loved each other and were comitted to each other, she relaxed a bit. But when she spoke of my boyfriend, she always referred to him as my husband. We lived together for five months and then decided that we should get married to make our families happy. At that point, my folks were elated and planned a beautiful wedding for us with five bridesmaids and all the rest. I wanted to become a nurse, and my husband is now putting me through college. That makes my parents realize we were mature enough to do what we did."

In sum, no matter how good living together may sound, there are problems. Guilt feelings are more prevalent than is commonly assumed. Instability of the relationship often causes the living-together arrangement to end much sooner than first expected by the couple. Because no legal documents bind the couple, and because there will be relatively little red tape should they decide to end their relationship, it is likely that *commitment* is de-emphasized.

Parental relationships are often harmed, sometimes beyond repair. Even where parents can accept their child's living with another person without marriage, they may wish it were not so and feel a sense of disappointment. Recall Kathy, who told us that her parents accepted her living arrangement, but that she knew how disappointed her folks were in her. While many people believe they have a right to do whatever will bring them happiness regardless of what others might think, many more are saying, "A few months of *playing house* is not worth causing parents anguish, or myself the hurt that is possible when things break up. If we love each other enough to want to be together, then we should love each other enough to commit ourselves to marriage."

8 marriage and the family

IN OUR SOCIETY most people do marry, for marriage is the *approved* relationship that allows a man and a woman to live together and to have sexual intercourse freely. In a year's time, there are approximately two and one-half million marriages taking place in the United States, compared to about one million divorces.[1] In spite of all the attention given to divorce and the breakdown of the family, marriage has been and continues to be very popular.

Recent research suggests that people generally are happy with their marriages. They feel that all the effort it takes to keep a marriage happy is worth it. It is well known that marriage is good for one's general well-being, for married people live longer than do single people and have better emotional health. It is also clear that marriage can bring happiness to people of any age—young, middle-aged, and elderly. It is not reserved for the young. Marital happiness need not decline with age.

Marriage is never without some conflict, however, if it is an intimate relationship. This is true in the happiest of marriages. The important issue is the manner in which this conflict is handled. Good communication is essential because it helps us better understand differences that can come between a husband and a wife. But even though some conflicts cannot be resolved, a marriage can be happy if we realize that in marriage we must also gracefully accept the things in each other that cannot be changed. Your chances for happiness, then, depend to a considerable degree upon your own willingness and ability to adjust to your partner. Changing your own way of thinking and behaving is never easy, but the more determined you are to have a happy mar-

riage, the more determined you must be to change when it is
required to make compromises. For example, suppose you
were brought up in a home where no one ever closed doors
or worried if Dad came into the bathroom to shave while you
were in the shower. Your marriage partner may have been
brought up in a home where privacy was the order of the
day. These two styles of living would require compromise on
your parts. You would have to respond patiently to your
partner's need for privacy and your spouse would have to
make adjustments to your desire for intimacy and dislike of
closed doors. To accomplish this would require that you
develop your skills in responding openly, freely, and honestly
to each other's needs. In marriage, you must remember to
concentrate not so much on your partner's behavior, but
rather on how you can make the relationship between you
and your spouse happy and strong. This is your responsibility
in marriage. Marriage is not a simple matter. Its requirements
for happiness include knowledge of your partner's needs
and personality, flexibility in dealing with changes and
adjustments, and the emotional maturity that will give
you patience.

*If a couple wants to get married and they think they are
ready, how can they really know for sure?*

No one can be *absolutely* sure. After all, marriage does involve some risk. Given the many factors that enter into an
intimate relationship, it is important that young people think
hard and long about the decision to marry. Are you mature
enough to handle the change from being single to the intimacy of a constant twosome? Are you economically prepared for this step? Is this someone that you want to spend
the *rest of your life* with?—for this is the intention with
which one should enter marriage. Can you handle quarrels
and conflict? Do you have similar values and aspirations?
    As John said, "A lot has to do with accepting and helping
and understanding the partner. Maybe you should think
about things you would be able to do without your partner—

things in which he could weigh you down. You may want to live alone a little before you get married to make more certain you are mature enough for this big step."

"To know if you're really ready for marriage, you must ask yourself a lot of questions and answer them honestly," suggested Janet. "If you are not honest with yourself, you will end up being more hurt than pleased. Ask yourself if you feel a sense of care, respect, and responsibility toward each other. Are you ready to settle down with him for *life?* If, after you are married, his job requires you to move to Africa, would you be willing to go with him? If you hear yourself questioning your love, then you are not ready. You must also ask yourself *why* you are getting married. If you are doing it just to get away from your folks or if you are getting married to show them that you are grown up, or to spite them, then you are getting wed for the wrong reasons. But if you know that you are getting married because you are mature and want to share your life with this man in order to bring him happiness and yourself contentment, then go ahead."

Unfortunately, education for marriage is left largely to chance and many young people marry with very little understanding of what is involved. Marriage is glamorized so much that young people often interpret a strong desire to go to bed as sufficient evidence that they are ready for marriage. They mix up sexual attraction and infatuation with love. Many teenagers have unrealistic expectations about the marriage relationship—that it is a bed of roses. Many marry with the idea that if it doesn't make them happy, they can always get a divorce. Thus we often see a lack of determination and commitment to stay married among teenagers.

If you are ready to get married, you will really want to make it work and so will your partner. You will recognize that you will not "live happily ever after" unless you work hard at it every day of your married life.

I would be very remiss if I did not suggest the usefulness of premarital counseling, particularly for people who are unsure of why they want to get married. A trained marriage and family counselor can be located by contacting a mental health clinic or a family-life agency in your community. You and your partner may be given tests to help you determine your own compatibility with each other. You may be counseled on how to improve your skills to get along with another person in the intimate, day-to-day world of marriage. This counseling will give you a much better idea of whether you are ready for marriage and whether you do have the right reasons for getting married.

Many family-life educators, divorce lawyers and judges, social workers, clergymen, legislators, psychiatrists, and sociologists like myself believe that premarital counseling would greatly reduce the number of unhappy marriages as well as the rate of divorce. Perhaps someday premarital counseling will be a prerequisite along with the other requirements that must be met to obtain a marriage license.

Does it make a healthy marriage when two people who have been going together since they were young get married? Or should they go out with other people too just to make sure, as some people say?

"When you are young, you should not date just one person," suggests Ted. "Rather, you should go out with many different people so you can compare what kind of boy or girl is good or bad for you in a relationship." Eighteen-year-old Rick said, "A long engagement is associated with a better marriage, but before you get engaged, it never hurts to be sure you have what you want by being able to compare your prospective mate with other steadies you have had in the past."

It is very clear to me that many married persons wish they had dated more before marriage. Looking back, they often feel that they may have missed something by devoting their attentions to one person and excluding all other possibilities. Many wish they had finished their education first, that they had had a chance to travel and to develop a better idea of what they wanted out of life. Quite a few also express their regret that they didn't get to know their partner better before marriage. When a person marries too young, or marries the first person he or she has ever gone with, after a few years many doubts arise.

June tells us what her mother had to say about the doubts she experienced after marrying June's father, the first and only man she ever went with: "Believe me, June, it is a mistake being in such a hurry to get married that you marry the first man who pays you any attention. I guess I did this because I was always fat as a child and my family teased me, so that I really felt ugly. I was sure no man would ever want me. I regret that I married very young right out of high school, with no chance to be on my own and enjoy my independence. I did not know myself very well, or what I really needed in a man to be happy. I was an uncertain person who needed someone strong to help me build up my self-reliance. Instead, I got a man who was no more confident in himself than I. Had I gone out with a few fellows before getting married, I think I would have found out more about what I needed in a husband. Your father and I never did get along—we couldn't agree on anything. I began to doubt myself as well as my choice of a husband. I doubted that we could have a happy marriage, and you know we didn't, because we are divorced."

June continues: "I wanted to go steady at sixteen, but my mother, thank goodness, persuaded me of the value of playing the field until I was older. I dated several boys in high school and when I met Bob, I knew he was the kind of person I could live with the rest of my life. Mother convinced me also of the value of not rushing into marriage as soon as I fell in love. She told me that if he really was the one for me and I for him, we would be willing to wait a few years for each other. If our relationship wasn't strong enough to withstand waiting until I was old enough for marriage, it surely wasn't strong enough to hold up a marriage. Now, at nineteen, we are engaged, and I feel very secure that we can have

a successful marriage. We are planning a wedding the summer
after we both graduate from college, which will be two years
from now. Although we know that dating and going steady
cannot give us a complete picture of what our marriage will
be like, we have given ourselves time to get to know each
other very well and to develop a sense of assurance that we
are right for each other."

Why do people get married?

Peter J. Stein, in his book, *Single*, has enumerated several
reasons why people might choose to marry. He says that the
main *pushes* toward marriage are: pressure from parents; a
strong need to get away from home; fear of independence;
loneliness; and guilt over still being single when society says
everyone should be married. Things that *pull* a person toward
marriage are: parental approval; desire for children; the fact
that all one's friends are getting married; a romanticized view
of marriage; physical attraction; need for love and companionship; desire for the security and social status that
marriage gives; and the idea of having a ready sexual partner.

While there are many reasons to marry, Stein also mentions some *pulls* toward remaining single: desire to pursue
a career and wanting the variety of experiences available to
a single person, such as being self-sufficient and the possibility of having an exciting life-style (along with increasing
sexual freedom); the freedom to change and move from job
to job or from place to place; and the sustaining of friendships that fill one's need for companionship.[2] When one
looks at the opportunities available to a single person, marriage for the teenager appears quite questionable. Although
most of us need to feel that we are terribly important to
someone else and that that person is totally dedicated to us,
marriage requires a commitment that many young people are
not ready to keep.

Sally illustrates the case of a typical teenage bride as she
says, "Now that we are married, the only time he acts interested in me is when he wants sex. He thinks his boyfriends

are just as important to be with as I am, and when he is not with them, he has them hanging around here. I thought I was going to be his one and only, but was I fooled."

Sally is expressing another basic reason to marry—to have a one-to-one relationship. We desire to be with that most important person who will give us emotional support, boost our self-esteem, give us affection and a feeling of respect, trust, and intimacy. How many young teenagers really are mature enough to give these things to a marriage partner?

People who are ready marry for companionship and unqualified love. They want to have someone around to talk with, to share common goals. They care as much for the happiness of their partner as for their own. They aren't thinking only of their own needs. Real love is reciprocal—that is, by giving love, one receives love.

Happiness is never guaranteed by a marriage certificate, but if we are happy persons, we will be happier in our marriage. Marriage between two persons ready for marriage will give them a peace of mind that can help the husband and wife fulfill each other's sexual needs. Sex will be beautiful—it will be an expression of love and trust. Marriage symbolizes sex with respect and love. Marriage in the above sense requires a maturity that is likely to be more developed as one grows older. Why not wait until you are in your twenties to marry when it can be more meaningful to you and, in the meantime, enjoy the many blessings of remaining single?

I am worried because I heard that teenagers have the most divorces. Why do marriages go wrong?

Records show that teenagers do have the highest divorce rates. Half of all teenage marriages end in divorce and the chances for a lasting teenage marriage are about one-third as good as for marriages of persons in their twenties.[3]

Marriages go wrong for many reasons. But teenage marriages seem to have their own special set of problems. One primary reason for the failure of many teenage marriages is that many young people use marriage as an *escape*. They escape from an unhappy family situation, from dependence on their parents, from having to become independent; or they might marry because everybody else is doing it. When people use marriage as a means of solving their personal problems, they may become very disillusioned and bitter upon discovering that marriage did not do what they had expected.

Another common reason for failure is that a teenage marriage limits a person's options for an education, for a better job, and better pay. "What fun can you get out of life," asks Bill, "when you never have enough money to buy the things you need to make you content. Sure, money isn't everything, but when you don't have enough to last from one payday to another, it can start lots of fights and unhappiness."

Sue mentions yet another major pressure on teenage marriage. "Divorce is higher for young kids because they haven't had the chance to satisfy individual needs (such as a career, traveling, recreational and emotional needs) before assuming the serious responsibility of marriage."

When you marry without knowing what you want out of life, it is almost impossible to satisfy your needs. Personalities clash when there is a wide gap in attitudes about the many aspects of marriage.

Teenagers who marry seldom know each other well enough to be able to make the compromises required in a happy marriage. When two people can't agree about having children, about how to rear children, or spend their income, on choosing the friends they are going to have around, on religion and recreation, how are they going to make marital adjustments? The fact of the matter is that teenagers, because of their youth and unrealistic expectations, do have more problems right from the beginning in establishing a happy marriage. Many do succeed, but more don't. It is a very risky business.

I love my boyfriend so much that I want to have his baby. Doesn't that prove that I am ready for marriage?

Today, having babies is not considered a prime reason for getting married. I can understand why you interpret your desire to have your lover's baby as proof you are ready for marriage. You are so emotionally involved with him that the thought of uniting your body with his in the conception of a child gives you the romantic feeling of being united in a deep bond of love.

But, you see, marriage is more than an emotional bond, and having a baby is not romantic. Physical desire that is part of loving is essential to having a happy marriage. However, as I said earlier, love, the kind that sustains a marriage, includes more than the physical urge to unite one's body with another. Real love includes the elements of caring, respecting, feeling responsible for the well-being and happiness of another person. Marital love is measured in part by how willing you are to change your own behavior to satisfy your partner's needs, how capable you are of talking to your partner about what you like and don't like about your relationship, including all aspects of your sex life. Marriage involves many practical things, such as saving money to pay bills and performing various household chores, as you know. Having a baby represents an awesome responsibility, and the desire to have one in no way assures that one is ready for parenting.

The college students I queried on this subject seem to agree with me. The girls answered this question with a resounding *NO*. Typical comments were: "You're not ready for marriage simply because you want to have his baby." "It sounds as though you are physically attracted to him but not emotionally involved. Reproduction is only one aspect of marriage."

Typically, the fellows said, "Make sure that 'having his baby' doesn't just mean *making love with him*. He should want a baby as much as you do, but remember that this should not be the main reason for getting married. It should be that you love him, that you care for and respect him, that you *both* are mature enough to care for a family."

Is love an important factor in the sexual relationship in marriage?

Love is the primary reason why most people marry. Sex is expected to be a part of the marital relationship. "To have

and to hold" as part of our marriage vow means just that.
Young people are often motivated toward marriage by their
strong physical attraction, as well as by their emotional
need to be together. But if sex is the only reason for a marriage, it will not last. No one factor is enough to make or
break a marriage. As Jeff has said, "Sex may be satisfying by
itself, but love enhances the act so much that I could never
say sex by itself is great. You have to have love to obtain the
greatest sexual enjoyment. Without love, you would not have
much of a marriage, with or without sex."

*How can you have a satisfactory sexual relationship in
marriage?*

According to many sexologists, the most enjoyable sex is
uninhibited sex. This kind of sexual response is not always
possible for an inexperienced girl or boy, however. It is difficult to achieve, too, when either the fellow or the gal has
unrealistic expectations or inadequate knowledge about
human sexuality and the joys of sex.

Terry, for example, thought all fellows knew exactly how
to perform sexually to give a girl the height of ecstasy. She
explained, "I expected my husband to be aggressive and to
take control of things. Instead, on our honeymoon he was as
uninformed about what to do as I. Our sex relations have
been disappointing until recently, but now we have been
reading a good book on human sexuality, and that has
helped. Things were a little mechanical as we began to try
things out for the first time, but last night everything was
beautiful and spontaneous. I had my first orgasm.

"It won't matter to us anymore who is assertive in sex—
him or me. We have learned that the important thing is to
warm each other up with kissing and petting until we *both*
want intercourse. And he understands that like most women,
I like to be held in his arms for a while after we are finished
and to be treated tenderly. We have learned a lot of things
about what each likes in sex, because we understand now
the importance of not keeping our likes and dislikes secret.
We have learned, too, never to go to sleep mad at each

other. Making up before we go to sleep often leads to love-making."

Terry is fortunate that she and her husband obtained the kind of sex information they needed to help them overcome some of the major problems people have in achieving a satisfactory relationship. Sexual inexperience on the part of the male or female will limit the pleasure that is possible from sexual intercourse. Every couple should read a good, authoritative marriage-sex manual prior to marriage.

Other things are important too. Cleanliness is essential, as we have mentioned in a previous chapter. A freshly showered body is most inviting. A smell of perfume might turn on a man. Some special cologne or after-shave lotion can enhance a woman's sexual arousal. Some men and women prefer making love in the nude. Others prefer that the woman wear a sheer, sexy nightie. I can't stress enough the importance of a clean, attractive body to increase the pleasure of sexual intercourse.

A girl often is inhibited sexually because she equates sex with shame or feels that her partner will not think she is a "good" girl if she is aggressive or uninhibited. Very many men have no idea of what women really like and yet won't admit they don't know everything about human sexuality. A clumsy man whose ego won't let him admit his sexual ignorance will not be a very satisfactory lover. A woman who believes a man just "naturally" will know how to please her is likely to find that her partner can't always guess her preferences and thus will think she has a very insensitive husband. In order to please each other, two people must *tell* each other what they want and expect.

Sam is a classic example of a husband who can be called a perfect lover. He tells about sex in his marriage: "I am twenty-three and have been married for four months. My dad was a good example for me. He taught me to be polite, kind, and sensitive to the feelings of others. I love my wife very much and she does not equate tenderness in my treatment of her with being "unmanly." When we make love we talk and whisper our love to each other. She tells me I make her feel like the most loved person in the world.

"We both enjoy foreplay done slow and easy. In fact, I get so much pleasure from feeling her responses to me develop that the act of intercourse sometimes becomes secondary to the foreplay. I begin our love play by kissing her mouth and the palms of her hands very tenderly and lightly. Then I move my hands all over her body, caressing her lightly at first and then massaging her breasts and thighs more rapidly and firmly. Sometimes we have oral sex and sometimes we masturbate each other. She knows how to excite me, too. She will gently stroke my penis with her hands or kiss and lick the tip gently at first. Then she will squeeze my penis real hard or suck on it. I love it when she gently scratches my back or kisses me on my nipples. We usually are ready for intercourse at the same time, but I always ask her.

"I know from my reading that a girl will be much more likely to have an orgasm if you continue the foreplay for twenty to thirty minutes. I also know that when I can last for fifteen or more minutes before I come, my wife almost always has an orgasm. However, she tells me she doesn't mind, either, when she doesn't come because she enjoys the closeness we share, which makes her happy with sex. So we don't have to play the game of pretend. My ego isn't shattered when I know she doesn't have an orgasm.

"Some of the most fun we have is when I surprise her during the day when she isn't expecting me to sweep her up in my arms and make mad, passionate love with her. She will surprise me, too, by teasing me at unexpected times. When she takes her clothes off and parades in front of the TV set, or steps into the shower with me, things happen. I hope we never lose the openness and spontaneity we now enjoy in our marriage."

Monotony need not creep into the sexual relationship if the couple will continue to put forth efforts to stimulate and interest each other. With time, some of the spontaneity will wear off, but then the couple will share a more relaxed enjoyment of sex. As a husband and wife grow older they may need more stimulation to achieve arousal. A wife may need to rub her husband's penis to help him get an erection—

but he will be able to last longer as he gets older, thereby increasing his wife's chance to have an orgasm.

Remember, the beautiful sight of a loving woman, a gentle word, a soft touch, a warm smile, a pleasant smell, can readily cause sexual arousal. A favorite dinner menu, a date out to dine and dance, even a single rose, can keep romance alive. Love, tenderness, talk, imaginativeness, cheerfulness, attentiveness, fun, humor are all key concepts useful in keeping sexual interest—romance—alive in marriage.

Do men feel the girl they marry should be a virgin?

This depends upon an individual's experiences and attitudes toward sex, love, and marriage. There is a positive aspect to not being a virgin at the time of marriage—intercourse immediately after marriage will not be as uncomfortable as it can be when the hymen is ruptured the first time by penetration of the penis. There may also be less awkwardness and fewer inhibitions when a couple already knows what each likes about foreplay and the positions that give them the most pleasure and satisfaction from intercourse.

Generally, I think that attitudes toward virginity are changing. College students seem far less concerned about the importance of wives' being virgins on their wedding night than their fathers were. "Hell no!" Dick exclaimed. "I'm a guy, and I'm not a virgin, so I don't expect my wife to be. After all, if she has had others, she won't be so curious and she can tell me how good I am!"

Ron said, "Men may say they prefer it, but realize it may be idealistic. If a guy loves a gal and wants to marry her, it shouldn't make much of a difference. To some men, it does matter, but most are cool enough to love the girl they plan to marry for what she is when they met, not what she was or did before they met."

"I read somewhere that high-school boys still think they want to marry a virgin," said Adele. "My brother, who is a high-school junior, says most guys say they don't because they don't want to be thought old-fashioned, but in reality

they still like the idea of marrying a virgin. If it's true that
more and more teenage girls are having sex, lots of guys will
be disappointed."

Most of the girls I queried expressed the view that a man
does not worry about this unless he is insecure about his own
manliness. Jan said, "If a man feels that a woman should be
a virgin, but that he should not have to be, then he is prac-
ticing the *double standard.* If men can have their pie, so can
women."

*Do you have to tell the guy you are going to marry that
you've had relations with another guy?*

Only if you think that your relationship will be better because of it—and only if he *really* wants to know. Very often
such knowledge can affect a relationship adversely—it becomes more of a releasing of guilt feeling for the woman than
a new basis upon which to build. This is an issue that has
both pros and cons. Do boys feel it necessary to tell their girlfriends all about their previous sexual experiences? Most girls
say it doesn't worry them. Why, then, is it important for a
girl to *confess all* to her boyfriend? It is essential that both
the boy and the girl love and trust each other enough to take
each other as they are with no anxiety about previous loves
or sexual experiences. A woman should ask herself what her
real motivations are for telling: to release her guilt by heaping
information on him? To make him jealous?

If a guy is real "macho" or immature, hearing about his
future wife's love life can create feelings of insecurity or dis-
trust. I know a woman whose husband kept asking, "If you
made love to others before we were married, how do I know
you aren't now?" This marriage was miserable while it
lasted.

If a couple truly feels that telling all will provide a new
basis for love and trust and they are mature enough to handle
this information, then what Charles says is valid: "I feel it
is important to the marriage's strength that the girl does
tell the guy if she did, but I can only say what I think. For

me, I feel it shouldn't matter if that previous love was real, but I would like to think she loved and trusted me enough to tell me."

Karl said, "I really don't see any reason for her to tell me. I am only interested in her from the time we began our relationship. What happened before is over and has no part in our life together. I don't want any thoughts or comparisons to creep into our love life. My girl was engaged before I met her, and she probably did have sex since she believes in it when you are in love. But now she is mine, so why go into the past? The past is dead."

Young women, too, have a variety of opinions on the subject. Janie believes "You don't have to tell the guy you are marrying that you've had relations with another guy. Usually he'll know. Personally, I think it's none of his business, but if he must know, and it bothers him not knowing, tell him the truth. If he really loves you, it won't make any difference in his feeling for you."

Sally added: "You don't have to tell the guy you are going to marry, but if you love and respect him, he should have enough love for you as you are, not for what you have done in the past. He shouldn't want to know, but if he asks, you should be open and honest, because if you can't be honest with him, then you can't be honest in marriage. It shouldn't make any difference what your past sexual experiences were to him if he really loves you."

We plan to get married right out of high school. What problems will we have?

Tom says it best: "Financial problems—I can just see them arguing over what she wants to buy and what he can afford. Since he is so young, he may want to spend money on recreation, and she may want to have a baby—wow!"

Financial problems often are overwhelming to a couple married straight out of high school, and the immediate restrictions placed on their activities could cause them to dislike one another. As Esther said, "I think they will resent each other for tying each other down. High-school students usually make less money than a person who goes on and gets some further training or education. When guys get married so young, they usually don't have a chance to increase their education. When you add money problems to the emotional problems that teenagers might have, you have a situation that can be very unhappy."

"Maybe it's how well prepared two people are to handle marriage that counts," suggested Leigh. "It surely depends upon how the couple can work out their financial problems and how willing they are to make sacrifices and forego luxuries they can't afford. If a guy waits until he is twenty-three or twenty-four, he will more likely be financially ready for marriage than with just his high-school education."

"On the other hand," Sandy added, "if you wait until you have enough money to get married, you might never do it. If two people are really determined to make their marriage work, maybe they can work out things better and faster together."

Sandy is being pessimistic when she suggests a couple might never marry if they wait until they have enough money. But it is perhaps better not to marry than to marry when you do not have sufficient funds to cover at least the *minimal* costs of a household. I believe that money is a major source of stress and breakdown of marriages—more so than sex. When a couple does not have enough money to afford the price of a movie after bills are paid, discontentment and disappointment with their marriage can enter the picture. Fighting and bickering over money can lead to violence and breakup of the marriage.

Carl is a young man who knows from his own childhood experience how destructive financial problems can be to a family. "If a guy is not well-off financially, he shouldn't marry," he said, "and I know from listening to my parents that a poor financial situation is a major cause of frustration and conflict. My folks fought so much about money—my father spent more than he made—that they finally got divorced. I had a hell of a family life listening to them fight all the time. I have some friends who got married right out of high school, and now three years later they are head over heels in bills, and they don't have any kids either."

Young couples should think seriously about their finances before they get married. If they are really determined to make their marriage work, financial problems need not be insurmountable. As Karen said, "Finances are a problem, but many times working out problems can bring you closer together—'Look what we can do together that we couldn't have done alone' is a nice feeling."

What sort of financial security is mandatory for the newly-wed couple?

At the time of marriage, it is important that the couple's income be enough to maintain a home and also to provide for the potential arrival of a child, even if it does not happen. Usually this is not the case in a teenage marriage unless they receive monetary help from their parents. Even when this kind of help is given, problems can arise. For example, the girl may accuse her husband of not being *man enough* to support her, thus tearing down his self-respect. Young people are often wasteful and know little about handling money. They tend to overspend, buy things on credit, and get so deeply in debt that separation often appears to be the only answer. When a person marries, he should be able to afford insurance—life, health, and household insurance. Often a job held by an untrained high-school student does not pay enough to afford even these essentials. And, unless a couple can arrive at some agreement about the questions of how and by whom the family income will be handled, they can run into all kinds of other snags.

It would be good if young people approaching marriage would consider all these financial issues first. "We will take care of trouble when it happens" seems to be the more common approach. Unfortunately, teenagers are often unable to handle such problems when they actually occur.

As a consequence, we have increasing numbers of divorces among couples who marry too young.

If a husband doesn't want his wife to work but they need the money or she wants to work, is this harmful to the marriage?

The college girls agreed that if they can't come to some mutual understanding about the wife working, the couple may find themselves getting into serious conflict. Anne was optimistic as she said, "If the wife wants to work until their finances are better, it shouldn't harm the marriage. It really depends on how important it is to the wife that she has the freedom to work if she wants to and on the reasons why the husband objects to her working. Both should be mature enough to realize when it is important that the wife work. In fact, it is only being realistic to expect that the wife may either want to work or will have to in order for a couple to have a satisfactory marital relationship." The traditional attitude that "the woman's place is in the home" is being discarded as both men and women are becoming more willing to exchange their roles.

I know a young couple recently married who have announced that he is going to take the responsibility for the cooking and housework and she is going to pursue her career as a physician. This young man obviously has no cultural hang-ups that cause him to feel less of a man because his wife has more education and a higher salary and work status than he. She is comfortable with the exchange of traditional roles, too, and furthermore, has too much invested in her career not to want and need to work as a doctor.

Jack commented, "Wouldn't it be silly not to realize the advantages of having two incomes? Eventually I plan to start my own engineering business and our double salary will get me there much faster. Martha would never be content without her career—and I realize that it is as important psycho-

logically for her to work as it is for monetary reasons. Men
should encourage their wives if they want to work. We have
agreed that when we have children we will have to come to a
mutual decision as to how much time she and I will give to
rearing them."

The fellows agreed that a wife's working could cause
more trouble than financial shortages if the husband can't
take not being the breadwinner. Tom said, "It's good for the
income, and the guy might learn to grow up. If the wife
works, she will increase her knowledge right along with him.
If the family needs the bucks, the husband will come to a
realization sooner or later that his wife should work."

Just as a wife should have the freedom to work she
should also have the freedom not to work if it is financially
feasible. The husband's financial situation should be discussed prior to marriage so that the wife who prefers not to
work because she considers marriage and child rearing a full-
time career will know that she can stay home. "I get very
angry," commented Ginny, "when I hear my mother apolo-
gizing to her friends for not having kept up her teaching
career. She did a beautiful job of caring for Dad and us kids
and I'm glad she didn't work outside the home! Women
should have the same right to choose not to work outside
the home as they do to work, and so should men."

Freedom of choice really is the issue. Ruthie felt that
a wife should have the freedom of choice to work whether or
not the money was needed. "I am getting a college education
so that I will have a degree, and the man I marry will be one
who agrees that I am free to work because that is what I
want to do. If he tried to impose his will on me, I would
know he is not the right man for me."

Ralph expressed a typical view of college men when he
said, "I expect my wife will work when we are first married,
to give us a good start. But when we have children, I hope she
will want to stay home and be a mother to them, at least
until the kids are in school all day. I believe that when a
wife works all day outside the home, she can become so
physically and emotionally fatigued that she will be irritable

with the children when she comes home. My fiancée will have a degree in nursing, which is just perfect for doing part-time work. Then she can arrange her schedule so she or I will be home when the kids come home from school and in the evenings. I know she has a strong desire to work at her chosen profession; she enjoys her work, and I will certainly want her to be happy. She has told me that working part-time while the children are young will be satisfactory for her."

That a wife will work is a very reasonable expectation, given the fact that the number of married women entering the labor market is increasing. According to a publication of the Population Reference Bureau, wives with children under six years of age have had a 56 percent increase in their entrance into the labor force since 1970. Childless married women under thirty-five have the highest worker rates of all married women. Over 44 percent of all married women are employed in the labor market. It also appears that when women have children, they leave the labor force temporarily. The same bulletin indicates that about seven percent of wives are earning more income than their husbands.[4]

Are marital problems caused when the woman is bringing home more money than her husband?

This depends on the man's ego. Tom, for instance, said that in his case, it wouldn't work out very well. "A man likes to feel that he is supporting his family," he said. "All his life, he has been brought up to think of himself as being the provider. It is a big part of his male image. It's the *macho* in him. He might like to have his wife bringing in some money, but to have her make more money than he, never."

Mike exclaimed, "It wouldn't bother me if my wife earned more than I! I would like it. Man, times are changing. I think a man should encourage his wife to excel in whatever she wants to do."

"I think it *can* work out if the man isn't made to feel guilty about it and is not being constantly reminded of it," said Marge. "My brother was married to a woman who made more money than he while he was working and still going to school. Unfortunately, she had a father who kept reminding her that the husband should *wear the pants in the family*. Eventually, she became very hostile to my brother. One day she went out and bought a new refrigerator, and when he asked her how come she hadn't even told him about her plans, she reminded him that since she was making most of the money, she didn't have to consult him. This really blew his mind. Eventually they were divorced. He could have taken her high salary, but *she* couldn't handle her *own* hang-ups about a husband's and wife's roles."

This bitterness is not always the case, however, as Tim tells us: "My mother just earned her master's degree in teaching and now makes more than my dad, who has an office job. He is so proud of her he brags all the time. They have always pooled their earnings, and it's never been *your* money and *my* money. Mother never reminds him that she is making more; in fact, we really don't think about it in our family. What is important is that Mom and Dad love each other and always take time to spend alone with each other. Every Friday night since I can remember, they have gone out to dinner and a movie or something by themselves. We have never resented her working. Dad and we kids divide up the chores so that she doesn't always have to be working when she is home. Our dad has taken care of us a lot, and I feel lucky for this, so Mom's working has been nothing but an asset for our family. She has worked since the beginning of their marriage, with the exception of time off when she had her babies."

Again we can see that attitudes of people involved have a great deal to do with how situations are handled. If a man feels comfortable, has a sense of self-respect, believes in a democratic family environment where husband and wife have fairly equal voices in decision making, he is not going to have many problems over the question of his wife's working or the size of her paycheck. Neither will the wife.

Should the spouse be forced to lessen his or her aspirations for fear of harming the other's ego? What about one's sense of self?

Unless one preserves one's own sense of self as being worthy and productive, it is unlikely that a person with high aspirations will be happy and contented. To be a happy spouse requires that one also be a happy self. Therefore, if one is forced to lessen one's own aspirations for fear of harming another's ego, one can become very frustrated, discontented, and unhappy. Eventually, the person whose ego is being spared may become a hated victim of the person who was forced to lower his or her aspirations.

Rather than to force another to forsake his or her aspirations or risk harming another's sense of self, it is better to look at marital roles realistically in the light of today's society.

Women work for various reasons. They may be trained or educated for a career and want to make use of it; they may have psychological needs to get away from the home environment (for example, they may not like housework and caring for children); they may genuinely love to work; and there may be a financial need for the extra money she can earn—which is the case more often than not. Mike was probably right when he remarked, "times are changing." Young people of today are very likely to expect that the wife is going to work at least during part of the marriage, and labor statistics indicate that almost three-fourths of all married women will work during part of their marriage.

We have discussed many reasons why people decide to marry, as well as situations that can cause a marriage to go wrong. Now we have questions that point to special issues that may cause problems, depending, too, upon the attitudes of the persons involved.

What adjustments must two people of different races make when they get married? And what about the children?

Persons of different races who marry must face the problem of prejudice. The degree of prejudice varies according to one's social background and environment. For example, if a person whose father is rich and famous or highly educated marries another of a different race, the marriage is likely to have fewer pressures against it than if the parents have middle or lower incomes. And, if a person marries another of a different race who is a well-known entertainer, the problem of prejudice seems to be less. Why? Money is power. Fame is power. Power helps insure that one's integrated marriage will be accepted by society. Who would slight actor Michael Caine, for example, whose wife is of a different race?

Many studies made on integrated marriages show that they are more readily accepted by the more highly educated and higher-income people of our society. Prejudice, that negative attitude toward various groups of people based on myth rather than fact, is learned, and with education it can be unlearned.

Although the problems of an interracial marriage, as in any marriage, depend on a variety of factors, and probably the most influential factor is the couple's social environment, other factors are important, too: parental acceptance, the personalities of the spouses, and the motives behind the couple's marriage.

Riva is a white woman married to a black man. Her problems, I think, are quite typical of an interracial marriage: "I was a graduate nurse on my first assignment when I met Ira. He was a medical assistant. I liked him for his looks and personality and was excited at the thought of dating a black man. But it was I who convinced him that we should go on a date. My parents hate blacks with a passion and I think I wanted to prove to myself that I did not have their prejudices, so I became involved with Ira as proof. At first, I liked the attention I got—I'm very, very blond and he's very dark. However, it ceased to be fun when we would be stopped by cops to prove *my* car wasn't stolen, or when someone shouted 'nigger lover' at me.

"Our relationship grew into a sexual attachment and before I knew it I was pregnant. He agreed we should get married. My folks didn't know about Ira, and I'll never forget their shock when I told them whom I was marrying and that I was pregnant. They refused to meet him or to come to our wedding. They wouldn't let my sister come to the church to be my maid of honor, either. The nurses at the hospital gave me a wedding party. Ira's mother was reluctant to accept our marriage, but she did come up from Louisiana to attend the wedding, saying she knew it would never work.

"Finding an apartment was a real hassle. I would look first and then arrange for Ira to look at it. When the landlord would see him, suddenly someone had just taken the apartment. We finally settled for a place in a part of the city much poorer than I had ever been in. I kept on working almost up to the day our baby was born. I was so worn out from nursing and doing all the housework and cooking that going to the hospital was like having a vacation. Ira never did help around the house, even after the baby.

"My most difficult time with prejudice was when our baby was born. The nurses at this particular hospital treated me like dirt. I heard one of them say how she just couldn't bear seeing a brown baby nursing on a white woman's breast. They gave me a minimum of attention.

"I wanted to show my beautiful baby to my parents and family so badly that one Saturday Ira drove me to my parents' home, let us out, and left, because he knew he was unwelcome.

"They let me in, and my mother, taking our son, said, 'Oh he is so light-skinned, he's quite pretty.' Timmy was three months old and quite irresistible, so that even my father began to respond to him. I was happy until Sunday morning. I came downstairs with Timmy and me all dressed for church. Mother looked at me, saying, 'Where do you think you are going with *that*—don't you think you have embarrassed us enough without advertising your shame!"

"I called Ira to come get me, and I cried. He was cussing *whitey* all the way home and at that time I agreed with him.

"About two months after this visit, I received a letter from my mother. She wrote, 'Look what you have done to our family. Your youngest brother refuses to attend school because the kids tease him so much about having a black brother and loving niggers that he can't stand it!' Was I at fault for this, or is it people's prejudice?

"Now that our child is of school age he is aware of parties to which he is not invited, and when he comes home crying because kids tell him he must have been rolled in the dirt when he was born, my anguish is difficult to handle.

"We didn't seem to be accepted as a couple by Ira's black friends, or maybe it's because I didn't want to associate with them. The nurses at my hospital ceased to invite us to their parties. We had a few white couples we saw now and then, but our social life got pretty sour.

"Eventually, Ira began spending most of his free time with his buddies and I was left to stay home with our child. He would remind me that I had instigated our relationship and got myself pregnant. His animosity toward *whitey* began to include me, and eventually our relationship deteriorated into violent fights, for we both have hot tempers. We are now divorced and I am taking a few extra courses to better myself in my career. Prejudice was not the only problem, but it certainly had a big part in the difficulties that we had."

As you can see, social prejudice, parental disapproval, temperament, and wrong reasons for dating and marriage were all a part of Riva's difficulties with her marriage.

Ray and Marcia, on the other hand, have had a successful, happy interracial marriage of three years. Although their story is probably an exception rather than the rule, several factors help account for the success of their marriage: they live on a large college campus where he is a star athlete; they have realistic notions about marriage; their reason for

marriage was love and the desire to be together. Ray is black.
Marcia is white. I asked them to tell me about the special
adjustments they've had to make as an integrated couple in
a racially segregated society.

"When we first met, we were completely unaware of
what the future held for us," explained Marcia. "We certainly
had not expected to marry a person of a different race. We
were both brought up assuming that we would each find
someone of our own race. The husband would work, the wife
would stay home and raise a family. Everything would work
out; we would never fight; we would have a wonderful love;
and our sex life would be perfect without effort—so went our
dreams.

"We had a surprise coming to us. We met each other one
summer night at a music college, and we knew we were attracted to each other. It was a little frightening. We just sat
and stared sneakily at each other for two months without
saying a word. Finally, Ray got up the courage to ask me to
go out to a baseball game, something that wouldn't force us
into an uneasy situation. Something clicked on that first
night. We developed an immediate warm friendship and later
a deep love for each other. We wondered day after day if it
would end, but it never did. That time never came, and a
year later, we were married."

Ray continued: "Togetherness, love, happiness, sex
that comes with marriage, were new to us. Since we were an
integrated couple, we thought we would have the added
problems of people making racial remarks or discriminating
against us. We wanted to be respected and loved for what we
were, like any other newlywed couple. Fortunately, we have
not had problems to the extent we expected, although we
know that in some parts of the country people are less
'tolerant.'

"In the first place, our parents approved of our marriage.
When I first brought Marcia home, my mother remarked
about whether I was aware of the problems I might have,
but she fell in love with my girl and soon forgot about any
racial differences. Her folks had brought her up to accept an

individual for the kind of person he is and not for the color of his skin. They lived by this principle, too, and accepted me right away. Her father is an avid athletics buff, and since I am a professional athlete, we struck up an immediate rapport.

"Neither our white friends nor our black friends had any problems accepting our relationship. We associate with several couples who are also integrated—but generally we have been accepted by all our family and friends.

"As stated earlier, we attend a large university in a large city. When we are on campus, no one seems to notice us. But that is not always true when we are out in public. I have a way to fix people though—when we are in a grocery store and some busybody begins to stare at us—I just look her straight in the eye and say, 'We are really human beings just like you.' That usually embarrasses them enough to make me feel good."

Marcia broke in: "But when some young dude made comments about me or about us when we were walking down the street, he used to get real mad and got into some bad fights."

Ray said, "I would just get so damn angry, all I could think of was to punch the guy out and make him apologize to this sweet, wonderful lady that I love. Now I have learned that there are ignorant people in the world and that I must always consider the source. Sometimes, even now, she has to hurry me away, though," he added.

Marcia continued, "We know many couples like us who do have trouble, and we don't know why we have not had many problems with prejudice. Maybe it's because of the warmth and sincerity we have between us that can be sensed at a distance. Maybe it's because our family and friends accept us and thereby shield us. Maybe it's because we are so committed to our marriage that we just won't let outside pressures affect it. No, our marriage is not much different from any other couple's, but we have some rocky roads to travel."

Marcia spoke of some of the problems they have faced— none of which are limited to interracial couples: "One of the main problems we have relates to Ray's being brought up thinking that he should take the lead role and be the bread-winner. I was to stay home and take care of the house. I had other ideas. I was brought up with a sense of independence and wanted to share the financial responsibilities. We had to work this out, talking for hours on end, fighting, and finally each trying to give in a little to the other. We decided to share. We both enrolled at the university. Ray had to get used to helping with the housework, something he had never done at home. I had to learn to take care of someone besides my-self. We work at little things in our marriage every day. We try never to have those silent wars like some couples we know have. We try to be honest with each other and get our feelings out into the open so we don't work up pent-up feelings of hostility.

"Communication is the most important thing in a mar-riage. We have to tell each other exactly what is on our minds. He can't read my mind, nor I his. I have to remember that I can't always have my own way, as I did pretty much with my folks. Sometimes he gets his way, and sometimes I get my way. We have learned how to compromise.

"Money caused us lots of trouble at first. Not only that we didn't have very much, both being students, but Ray was a spender and I was a saver. Eventually we came to grips with the situation. He has learned to save money a little more, and I have learned to be more reasonable about spending money. We still fight once in a while about money, but when Ray wants to buy that album, he thinks twice, knowing that I want to save for school next year. When I want to forget about going out on Saturday night, I think about how im-portant it is to our marriage to have some fun and recreation together."

Ray and Marcia both agree that they have a good sex life. "We both had similar values, but both being a little selfish, had to learn to think more about each other's needs. What-ever happens, we try to make the other feel good about it and not feel like a failure because sex isn't always perfect for us. We know we won't always have good sex. Factors such as being tired from work or being emotionally upset about this or that will enter the bedroom with us. Having a good marriage without sex would not be acceptable to either of us; having sex without a good marriage would be a farce.

"Interracial marriage—we really don't know what that means, but to love another person the way we love each other, we do know about," they concluded.

The happiness of a marriage is never determined by any one factor, as Marcia and Ray have so beautifully illustrated. Many of the *pluses* in their marriage include approval of their relationship by family and friends, a deep love and abiding commitment to make their marriage work, personalities that are similar in terms of similar values, the willingness to compromise, and knowledge of what makes a successful marital relationship. Racial differences are not necessarily a barrier to marital happiness when the couple understands what they are doing.

What problems would two people have when they are of different religions?

The general public as well as religious institutions seem to accept interfaith marriages more readily these days. Many men and women who are of differing faiths invite their pastor, rabbi, or priest to perform their wedding ceremony jointly.

Of course, some parents still do object to their child's marrying outside of the family's religious faith. Many of them fear that when this happens there will be a strong tendency for their child eventually to drop out of their church. This is a legitimate fear, perhaps not so much in terms of keeping up membership in a particular church, as a fear that their child will no longer value religion. In the same way, certain religious institutions object to interfaith marriages. They may be more concerned about keeping their membership intact than they are in helping people maintain a high value for religion.

Religion can be a very positive force toward achieving a happy marriage. Studies show that people who have a strong religious faith and participate as a family in church activities usually have a much better chance for a long, happy marriage. Religious pressures exerted by family and religious institutions can also create a negative force, however. Avoidance of problems depends to a great degree upon the strength of a couple's love and commitment to each other.

From my studies and research, I believe that it is far more important for the husband and wife to value religion to the same degree than it is for them to belong to the same religious faith. As Liz said, "I feel very strongly that my children should go to religious school and that we all should attend church regularly together. My husband doesn't really care if he ever sees the inside of a church. We were both brought up in the same church, but we fight about religion all the time."

Rod explained that he was brought up in a home where his father was Catholic and his mother Protestant. He grew up feeling very much a part of both churches, although he was baptized Catholic. "My father was president of the men's club of mother's church, and they were both active in the couples' club so that many people didn't even know that Dad wasn't a member," he said. "Mom participated equally in the activities of Dad's and my church. We never had any arguments over religion. Religion was very important to both my parents and to us kids.

"My sister isn't as fortunate though. She married a guy who belongs to the Lutheran church and his parents hassle her all the time about whose church the children should be baptized in. They agreed before they were married that since my sister would be the one to take them to church, it should be up to her. It's too bad that Sis is having such bad in-law troubles. They will hardly speak to her, and Dick has just about told his parents to let them alone or they won't see them very often."

Religious issues are best resolved, of course, before the marriage. It is important to talk to your intended mate about your religious values and discuss how you feel about church membership and participation. If you belong to different religious faiths, decide exactly what you will do about the various issues involved.

When should a couple decide to have a baby, and what should go into making this decision?

Having a child can be a beautiful expression of two people's love for each other. But, as I said earlier, the decision to have a child involves much more than an expression of love. Are you ready to take on the awesome responsibility of bearing and rearing a child? Are you mature enough to combine your roles of mother and father with those of husband and wife? Once a baby is born, it will require your attention twenty-four hours a day, which means you will have far less time to give attention to your spouse. You will have to make many changes in your life-style, which can be disruptive to a marriage if you have not thought through the reality of having a child. Daily routines will be changed—your sleeping habits, your eating schedules, your social life. There will be less money in your pocketbook, due to the added cost of another family member.

Having a child when you are knowledgeable about, and prepared for, the responsibilities and changes that a baby will bring into your life can be a most happy, fulfilling experience. Children bring much joy to a marriage when they are planned for and wanted. But, I must stress the importance of *waiting* to have children so that you can give your marriage a chance to work smoothly, free of pressures. There is no rush to have that first baby, for medical science has made it very safe for a woman to have her first baby when she is in her thirties. People are living much longer, so even if you wait several years to have children, you can be assured a good chance to see them grow into adulthood.

One should always make the decision to have a child with careful planning. As Alice said, "When a couple is financially as well as emotionally ready, then they should think about having a baby. They should both be sure they know each other well, and they should both want a child. Taking care of a baby requires much knowledge, patience, and time. Usually a couple is not emotionally mature enough or financially ready until they have been married a couple of years. There should be time to adjust to each other first."

Ralph added, "A couple should realize the changes in their lives and activities that a baby will bring and make sure they are ready for these changes. It is important that this decision be mutual and that the income be enough to support the extra expenses. If the wife works, plans should be made about when or if she will return to her job."

Ralph brings up another important matter. Three cannot live as cheaply as two, and babies do cost money. According to a publication of the Population Reference Bureau, in 1977 it cost in the range of from $31,675 (in a low-cost-plan, nonfarm family) to $53,830 (in a moderate-plan, nonfarm family) to raise a child to the age of eighteen.[5] (This does not, of course, include the subsequent cost of a college education, which would add another twelve thousand dollars, according to 1977 prices.) Most of these costs are spent on food, housing, and transportation.

Most young women and men believe it is good for a woman to work after marriage and start building up her work rights for seniority, retirement, and the like, or her career before kids arrive. In that way, it won't be so difficult for her to return to her work place should she want to or have to later on.

One should always consider the question of what might happen to a wife's career if she should have children. It is also important to point out here that a wife's working is not harmful to the children per se. Studies of children whose mothers work outside the home show that, whenever adequate child care is provided, there is no difference in personality and intellectual development from children whose mothers do not have a job. Many students have told me their mothers worked while they were growing up, but that their mothers spent as much time with them as the

nonworking mothers of their friends did with them, at the
time when it really counted—in the morning and after dinner
until bedtime. They felt they grew up a little faster because
of the added responsibilities they had. Mamie, for example,
explained, "We older children had to help the younger ones
get dressed and ready for school or to go to the baby-sitter
while Mom made breakfast and got herself ready to leave for
work. My brother and I helped with the housework and
learned how to cook at a very early age. I used to get angry
when I couldn't always go out and play with the kids, but I
appreciate now how much more I got out of life, learning to
be self-reliant and how to take care of myself and others as
well."

   A mother need not fear she is neglecting her children
or harming their psyche when she has an outside occupation.
Many other factors influence a child's development, such as
how supportive the child feels his parents are of him, the
kind of child care provided in the parents' absence, attitudes
of parents toward their children, the type of discipline used
for children, and general social environment. But whether or
not a wife will return to work is another decision that should
be considered prior to having a child.

What roles should a man and woman have as parents?

The most important role played by parents is to relate to
their child so that he or she will grow up feeling loved, independent, and emotionally secure. This requires that parents
give their child support, acceptance, and discipline.

   In our society, nurturing traditionally has been the task
of the mother. Father was considered the disciplinarian. Fortunately, this role stereotyping is being shattered by today's
parents as they share all the family roles. Such sharing of
roles can only be healthier for everyone in the family circle.
It is important that fathers share the nurturing role so that
when little Johnny comes running in the house with a cut
finger he will be just as likely to cry, "Where's Daddy" as
he will "Where's Mommy." Fathers need the opportunity to

establish a warm relationship with their children, and I think
it is great for the families of the future that men are sharing
this nurturing role with their wives.

In the same way, mothers are sharing the role of disciplinarian, as they have always done to some extent. When
rewarding children for good behavior and punishing them
firmly with love and consistency for bad behavior, mothers
are sharing a crucial role in helping their children learn to accept responsibility for their own behavior and to respect the
rights and feelings of others.

College students have repeatedly expressed their desire
to share family roles when they get married. For example,
Cynthia feels that the father should help care for the child
from birth on. "He should share experiences with his child
and not leave the bringing up of the child to its mother,
as so often happens. He should be firm but patient with his
children," she says.

"A father should be kind, loving, and responsible," said
Rick. "He should teach his sons to express affection and to
express their feelings when they are hurt, as well as teaching
them to be strong. He should show affection to his daughters,
also, and help teach them to be strong, independent, and
confident women. He should make sure that his children have
enough food and clothes and shelter to grow up healthy and
happy."

Sharon exemplifies the feelings of many college women
as she says, "A woman should share experiences with her husband, and *together* they should raise their children. A mother
is more of a comforter; in our society, she is around more to
help her kids through any crises. She is more active in children's social activities. She is responsible for taking care of
their clothes and seeing that they eat a proper diet. She
should discipline her children when they do something that
warrants it and not wait for the father to come home. But
Dad should be *very* much involved in deciding upon the discipline that will be used."

"I think that mothers are more prepared to bring up children than are fathers," added Rick. "But men can learn to

become good fathers. My dad got custody of me and my two brothers, and he has been considerate, understanding, and fair in his discipline. He is a damn good cook, too, although we all pitch in and help."

Kim suggested: "I think it is a good idea for husbands and wives to share and exchange their roles—they will learn to appreciate each other more. A man should know that a woman's role is not just child care and housework. A woman should know that a man's role is not just breadwinner and disciplinarian. Then, if a separation should occur, each would be better able to handle the role left vacant by the other's absence. Parenting is an awesome responsibility. The parents' main duty is to provide their children with a firm home base, a place where a child knows he is loved and welcome.

Much more can be said about marriage and the family, but these words from *The Prophet* by Kahlil Gibran perhaps sum it up best:

> Love one another, but make not a bond of love:
> Let it rather be a moving sea between the shores of your souls.
> Fill each other's cup but drink not from one cup.
> Give one another of your bread but eat not from the same loaf.
> Sing and dance together and be joyous, but let each one of you
> be alone,
> Even as the strings of a lute are alone though they quiver with the
> same music.
> Give your hearts, but not into each other's keeping.
> For only the hand of Life can contain your hearts.
> And stand together yet not too near together:
> For the pillars of the temple stand apart,
> And the oak tree and the cypress grow not in each other's shadow.

As one student said about marriage, "It is growing separately, together."

9 what about homosexuality?

TEN YEARS AGO students were quite reluctant even to discuss homosexuality. Now they are willing to talk about it and to ask questions. From what is being conveyed through these questions, however, it is clear that most teenagers (and probably most of the adult population as well) are very ignorant about the subject.

Just what is homosexuality?

Homosexuality may be defined as a person's sexual *preference* for another of the same sex. A homosexual girl (a lesbian) will fall in love with another girl, and if that other girl is also a homosexual and reciprocates her feelings, the two may enter into a loving relationship.

In discussing typical characteristics of homosexuals and their relationships, it is important that one does not make sweeping generalities. Each homosexual is an individual with his or her own unique personality traits and experiential make-up. Each homosexual relationship takes on its own characteristics. However, from talking with both male and female homosexuals and reading the literature, it seems that some broad truths can be pointed out.

According to Arno Karlen, in his book *Sexuality and Homosexuality*, most lesbians relate to others similar in age and social background. Some girls just meet occasionally to express their sexual needs, while many others set up a partnership in which they live as two married persons would. One of them may play the male or *butch* role, though this is not a necessary element in the lesbian relationship. One may wear a more masculine type of clothes and may even bind her breasts to flatten them. Her main role may be that of the breadwinner and the aggressor in sex. The other partner may play the feminine role and dress and behave in the *typical* female way. She may become completely dependent for support and protection upon her partner, and she may include in her role that of housekeeper. However, many lesbians play no definite "male" or "female" role, and sometimes there is a mother-child or sister-sister type of relationship with no sex between the two partners.[1]

A homosexual male usually will become attracted to another male fairly close to his age and is likely to have a strong desire for sexual contact. Often the relationship is one in which the two male homosexuals have occasional sexual relations on a dating basis.[2] The recently published report *Homosexuality: A Study of Human Diversity*, by Alan P. Bell and Martin S. Weinberg, which reports on the latest investigations by the Kinsey Institute for Sex Research, states that homosexuals are no more or less sexually active than are heterosexuals.[3] While men generally are more interested in impersonal sexual encounters than women, many male homosexuals, like their lesbian counterparts, live together in a close partnership in which they set up housekeeping and may live in many ways as a married couple. However, the average male homosexual affair lasts three to four years; the average lesbians' about six years. And, like lesbians, male homosexuals do not always divide up typical male-female roles. They both will play the aggressive and passive roles in their sex relationships. They will usually share all expenses, as both partners will most likely have jobs and feel equally responsible for their partnership.[4]

I wonder what it would be like to discover you are a homosexual. How do they handle this discovery?

Sexual preference as expressed in homosexuality is only *one* part of a person's total personality. But the way society views the homosexual can put great stress upon him or her and bring about emotional problems. What would you do if you had been a star football player in high school, received good grades in school, were an honor student and a generally like-able guy, and then after realizing that you liked boys instead of girls, found that your society views you as a criminal, a pervert, a molester of little children? Would this bother you? What if you had to live all your life keeping your homo-sexuality a secret from your family and close friends because you feared if they ever found out they would want nothing to do with you? Or that you would lose your job if your sexual preference were discovered, no matter how well quali-fied you might be? I asked nineteen-year-old Gary to tell me how he coped with this dilemma:

"Life can be a real drag at times, just as for the hetero-sexual, and other times it can be all worthwhile. A fear of letting friends know of my homosexuality, especially while I was in high school, was a constant problem. At age sixteen or seventeen, people really don't know much about homosex-uality except that it's different. It poses a threat to them, and they feel that associating with a gay person will subject them to ridicule—as it does. It's terribly aggravating to try and hide your secret from close friends for fear of rejection and harass-ment—as I have experienced.

"Because high-school friends found out, I went through a lot of hell my last year at school. Putting up with name calling and snickers upset me so much that I began to skip school and no longer took part in many activities. If you think going to the locker room was easy, forget it. Other guys can be such asses that you begin to feel nothing is worth the harassment. But I couldn't change how I felt. I began to drift away from school friends because I withdrew from activities, and soon I found some real friends at a gay bar. Then life seemed worthwhile again. I began to do things with other gay people and really felt good about myself. I felt I had made the right decision and really knew what I wanted. I wanted to be myself—I was a person who preferred other young men as friends and lovers to having girlfriends.

"What I really hate about my life is that it's so confining in contrast to my personality—confining in the sense that I can't be myself whenever I feel like it. Not being able really to be together with my homosexual friend—walking down the street holding hands, being together at dinner in a restaurant—has and always will bother me. I hate trying to hide my affection for my lover in public, but it is impossible to avoid disregarding other people's reactions. It would cause too much hassle to let people ever know about us, let alone show others we love each other very much.

"Homosexuals have their problems just as any other group of persons who are discriminated against—blacks, Indians, poor people. During high school, I got so sick of *fag* jokes from others I could have screamed. I think it takes so much stamina to put up with ignorant people that all gays should be commended for this alone.

"As for what I would like to be as a person, I am not sure. At this point, I am happy and satisfied with my life. Sometimes I catch myself thinking about how nice it would be to be a heterosexual male. Not for sexual reasons, but for the convenience of it, being able to go anywhere and be yourself in front of strangers. To be honest, I am too emotionally involved with my present lover to even think about changing. I'm happy and intend to live day by day, not fretting about what will happen to me in the future. Other people seem to worry about my sexuality, but I don't."

How many homosexuals are there?

It is speculated that there are between two and four million homosexuals in the United States.

I have heard from some fellows that they can always tell when a guy is gay. What should you look for?

Avoid making judgments about someone's sexual preference based on appearance. Looks are very deceiving. Relatively few homosexuals live up to their ugly stereotypes.[5] Homosexuals come in both sexes and in all ages. They may be blond, gray, brunette, red, bald, bleached, curly, or straight-haired individuals. You find them among all professions—football, basketball, and baseball players, bankers, clergymen of all denominations, teachers, nurses, bus drivers, hair stylists, ditch diggers, college professors, factory workers, and your own best friends. Homosexuals grow up in rich, poor, and in-between families.

As Alice said, "Many men who are not sports-oriented and look well groomed are labeled gay. Men who have big physiques are never taken as gay, and they could just as well be. Anyone could be gay, and it cannot be determined on appearance. There are no particular traits. A guy I saw who was very effeminate turned out to be one of the *sexiest* men I ever dated. 'Judge not, less ye be judged,' is a good policy. I have met guys whom I never suspected, and it turned out they were gay. Nice guys, too."

"There is no real way to tell if someone is gay," said Sam, "unless they tell you or make a pass at you. They are the same as anyone else except for their sexual preference." Roy expressed another view, however: "Usually a homosexual will stand out like a sore thumb. His style of dress, his mannerisms, his voice, his hobbies will tell you."

In all honesty, the way a minority of male homosexuals behave and dress appears to have given quite a few young people the idea that all homosexuals behave in a rather bizarre manner. I have many gay men and women among my friends who do not fit this unfortunate stereotype, and the majority of homosexuals are ordinary in behavior and appearance. One's sexual preference does not constitute one's whole personality, as I have said before. Furthermore, just as a heterosexual person's preferring the opposite sex is *normal* for him or her, so also a homosexual person's preference for the same sex is *normal.*

But what about the minority who do fit the stereotype? Why do they act like this?

Those homosexual males who dress in a so-called feminine manner—wearing jewelry, brightly patterned silk shirts, tight pants, high heels, and outlandish hair styles are often doing this as their means of getting back at the straights in our society. If it angers other men to see them appearing in this fashion, flaunting their sexuality around, the homosexual male has perhaps been able to relieve some of his animosity and hostility toward the nonhomosexual world, which is filled with prejudices and discriminatory practices.

Listen to what Nancy has to say about three of her co-workers: "I am a beautician, and when I was married, I invited all the people in my beauty shop to attend. Three of my coworkers were male homosexuals—and they were hostile toward heterosexual males and often took delight in putting them down by acting out the stereotype. Knowing that my husband-to-be and his brothers were all *macho-type* athletes and hostile to homosexuals, I asked my three friends to come to the wedding and reception dressed in regular slacks and shirts. They did, although their shirts were in brightly colored silks. At the reception held in our home my three friends chatted with others, enjoying the food and drinks. That is, until my brothers-in-law began talking in loud voices about the fun they had punching out *queers*, and other such derogatory comments. Two of my coworkers who were lovers picked up on these comments and before long they were deliberately *swishing* around the room, and began to show signs of their affection. The third gentleman saw the predicament I might be in and quickly talked the other two into leaving before any incident took place. Nothing would have occurred if my relatives had been on their good manners, for they all knew that my three male coworkers were homosexual."

Can you tell if a woman is a lesbian by the way she dresses or acts?

You really can't tell lesbians by appearance or behavior, either. In this day and age, both nongay women and lesbians wear male and female styles of clothing. As in the case of a male homosexual, unless a lesbian reveals herself, her secret is well kept. Women are allowed to behave affectionately toward each other and they can embrace and dance together in public. And this kind of behavior usually is not suspected as homosexual when performed by women.

I heard that many years ago homosexuality was not considered as bad as it is today. Is this true?

Although homosexuality in more recent times has been labeled as deviant behavior and deemed immoral by religious and legal bodies, it has existed all over the world and through all time. When you look into historical data you find that early civilizations approved homosexuality. It was practiced by the ancient Babylonians and Egyptians. The Greeks believed it was as normal as, and more tender than, heterosexual love, and it was also a very popular practice among the Romans. Socrates, Alexander the Great, and Julius Caesar were some of the more celebrated homosexuals.

Religious history, according to Karlen, indicates that when society was matriarchal—that is, headed and run by women (who were sometimes thought to have supernatural power)—homosexuality was treated as a *normal* kind of behavior. Then, when society changed to worshiping the authoritarian male god and men became the *rulers* of the family, homosexuality became equated with ungodliness and was considered morally wrong.[6] The early Jews were preoccupied with survival as a people, which led them to denounce homosexuality in very severe terms. Men were required to have sex with women to bear children and increase the species; homosexual behavior does not, of course, result in population increase. This denunciation of homosexuality as unnatural continues to be fostered by various religions.[7]

How does a person become a homosexual? Is it really a sickness as I have read?

There are many theories about the causes of homosexuality. Michael Schofield, a sociologist and author of *Sociological Aspects of Homosexuality*, has concluded that it is a great mistake to think that homosexuals are sick just because some doctors consider homosexuality a neurotic condition.[8] The anxiety that grows from a homosexual's fear, anger, frustration, and stress can cause anyone to become emotionally ill. But to assume that all homosexuals are sick because some are unable to withstand the social pressures that cause their anxiety is preposterous, don't you agree? This assumption by psychiatrists grows out of the fact that the homosexuals they know are their patients. The public goes along with the definition of homosexuality as a sickness because no one is able to say for sure what it is or how it is caused.

Some who have studied homosexuality, such as C. A. Tripp, suggest that it can start from purely physical association.[9] Boys are usually interested in their bodies and tend to explore their genitalia at an early age. When they discover their penis, they are likely to begin to masturbate. Enjoying and liking his maleness, a male can develop strong sexual desires toward other men. In situations where men are segregated, the likelihood increases that a man will play out homosexual tendencies.

You have probably heard about Sigmund Freud. He felt that our sexuality was inborn, that it was a matter of instinct. Others who have studied sexuality believe that whether we are a heterosexual preferring the opposite sex, a bisexual enjoying both sexes, or a homosexual preferring the same sex, our choice may be more a matter of social forces than biological forces. For example, a boy who is weak or awkward and is made to feel shy or ugly may think himself unworthy of ever gaining the love of a woman when he grows up. A person who feels insufficiently masculine by social standards may desire not to compete for favors of the opposite sex and may develop a preference for men.

In doing research on homosexuality, I have found that familial upbringing seems to present an inclination toward homosexuality. Bob, for example, a nineteen-year-old college student, presents almost a classic case. He told me his mother always tried to make a girl out of him to replace his sister, who had died at birth. "She kept me in long curls until I started school, and I was never allowed to play with boys for fear I would get hurt," he said. "Even now I have to call her to let her know I won't be in at a certain time, or she will begin to worry about me and call my friends or the police to find me. My father is just the opposite. He yells at me and never gives me credit for anything. I don't think he would care if I just dropped dead. Now, I can't stand to have women wanting sex with me. I think of my mother, and I get sick of the thought of having sex with a girl. I enjoy being single, and I enjoy making love with men. I enjoy being independent and responsible just for myself. Marriage is out for me because I have never seen anything good about it after living with my mother and father."

Rachel is another example of a homosexual with an unusual family background. She hates her father with a passion and feels bitter toward her mother. "All I have heard from my mother is that if it weren't for me she wouldn't have had to marry my bastard father. He is a terrible man—drinks all the time and then comes home drunk to beat her. Then she takes it out on me. When I was just a little girl she would punish me by threatening to leave me with him and would force me to pack her suitcase. I can remember always being afraid that she would leave me with him. He is an evil man, and many times he would come into my room at night and try to touch my *privates*. The thought of having sex with a man now is terrifying. I hate men. Now that I am eighteen, I have found happiness with a very kind woman who is about ten years older than I. We don't have any sex, but sometimes I really feel as if I want to have contact with her body. Maybe we will some day. She has taken me in to live with her and doesn't seem to mind that I can't do much about sharing expenses while I am in college."

Cindy, another lesbian, examines her background and begins by saying, "You know it's funny when people laugh and joke about sex, but it's not funny when you are a homosexual and feel you must laugh the hardest when jokes about *queers* and *gays* are told. It is very difficult for me to talk about my condition. I fear discovery and mockery so much.

I think I have always had homosexual tendencies. I think it only required the right time, place, and person for them to *unveil* themselves.

"My family life was not pleasant. My father worked in a dull factory job and often came home frustrated and would take out his frustration on me. Rarely a week would go by that I wasn't hit. I learned to hate my father—hate him with all my being. My mother felt sorry for me, but she loved my father and wouldn't do anything against him. I could never talk with my parents, for everything I would say only seemed to bother them. Sex was never talked about. I learned how to masturbate when I was seven years old. I discovered that masturbation was a very pleasant experience. It removed me from my immediate surroundings for a short while. I did it every time I could, for I could forget my problems for that short while. But one day my mother caught me, and she was so shocked that she couldn't even speak. Then she told my father, and I got a terrible lecture from my father on what a terrible, terrible thing I was doing. I tried to stop but after a while I just couldn't keep from doing it; but I made sure my mother wasn't around.

"All through school I felt terribly lonely. I felt dumb and ugly and of no worth to anyone. I spent all my time convincing myself that I would always be alone. I didn't like boys, and I never had dates. I hated school, and then one day I was introduced to an out-of-school, all-girl organization. I was very comfortable with these girls. I was accepted. I felt good. I leaned on my female friends to protect me from the outside world. At the age of sixteen, I met a very strong, protective girl, and I had my first homosexual experience. I wasn't too ugly to be loved after all. She made me feel so important. I loved her. She excited me. When we embraced, I felt a sense of security I had never before known. But somehow some of our friends began to catch on to what was happening between us. These pressures and threats to tell our parents broke us up. I am not sorry for this beautiful relationship. I hope I will find someone to love and be loved by again."

I do not want to leave the impression with you that all lesbians hate their fathers. Rhonda had a very loving relationship with her dad. "I have fond memories of Dad, who always had time to read to me or to play games. He died when I was thirteen and now at nineteen I still think of him often.

"My mother always seemed to resent the attention Dad gave me. She was demanding of me, always blaming me for everything the other kids did. After Dad died, she started chasing around, and then, being the oldest, I had to take care of everything. One of her favorite ways of punishing me if she caught me slapping one of the kids for being bad was to grab my hand and start to force it down over the gas flame until I screamed for mercy. She never did put my hand into the flame, but I never knew that she wouldn't.

"Now I don't even want to think of myself as a woman. When I fell in love, it was with a girl younger than I. She moved into my apartment and I am enjoying the *husband* part of our relationship. I work and she stays home and plays housewife. Our sex life is not divided into any sex role types. Sometimes she's the aggressor. Sometimes it's me."

Gary is convinced that his family upbringing is the cause of his homosexuality. "I wish I had been closer to my father, for now I know I never will be, even if I have the chance to try. Sometimes I think I was not given a fair deal. My mother can't understand why I am gay, although we never talk about it.

"About the only really happy times I can remember with my father occurred when we lived in Texas. My father owned horses, and he would let me ride them with my friends on special occasions. In 1968 we moved to the midwest and my father remained in Texas. Ever since then my sister and I have lived with my mother, and we have seldom seen our father except on an occasional weekend or a holiday. Mother has been the breadwinner, disciplinarian, teacher, and friend, all by herself. I am not close to my father at all. Even when he does come home, I can't bring myself to look him in the face when I talk with him. Maybe this was one of the reasons for my becoming a homosexual. One always hears of the overprotective mother, and I surely have one. I never did things like play football, baseball, or learn to fight for myself as other boys do from their fathers. As far back as I can remember, I always went places with my mother and sister. I have two aunts and six girl cousins we associated with. I was not, and still am not, exposed to anything but women and their interests in our family life.

"But what I want to do with my life is not particularly associated with femininity; I want to become a veterinarian. I have always loved animals and have many of them myself. I laugh at the myth about gay men all being dancers and hairdressers. I like to dance, but I would never make the professional scene, and I can't even imagine myself becoming a hairdresser. It's funny how so many people believe we can't do or want to do anything but work that is considered women's work.

"I have never had any guilt feelings for anyone except my mother—and then only occasionally. I'd think about how hard she tried by herself to raise me and how much she loved us and all the things she did for me. I have gotten over these feelings but still don't talk about them with her. I figure, why should I feel guilty for being what I am and have to be right now."

These five cases show the kinds of family conditioning that are known to exist in the backgrounds of many homosexuals. However, we must not forget that many children grow up in similar circumstances and do not become homosexual. We must then conclude that environment is not the only determining factor.

Research by endocrinologists suggests that homosexuality may be a matter of biochemical conditions existing at birth. Jim, for example, had a wonderfully happy childhood with loving parents and brothers and sisters. Yet he remembers the dreams and fantasies he had when he was a very young boy about various men. When he was eleven, he felt certain there was something different about himself. He seemed to have feelings toward boys that his friends had toward girls.

Now that he knows he is a homosexual, he says that he believes he was born that way.

Harold, too, thinks he was born to be a homosexual. He had a very positive family background. "My parents were very loving and I was and still am very close to them," he recalled. "I am the middle son of seven boys and the only one who turned out to be gay, so it must be biological. One brother is a priest, another a plumber, and I'm a pharmacist.

"I think I have known I was different since I was about four years old. I can remember a particular experience around that time. I was playing with dolls and would make them real sexy—tearing off their clothes and making sexy swimsuits and the like. I would have my girl dolls kissing each other, and one day as my mother was watching me, she started to cry. 'Oh, Harold, I don't want you to grow up and be a homosexual.' I asked her what that meant and she told me, 'It is like when a man likes another man the way I love your dad.' And I couldn't figure out what would be wrong with that, and I still don't find anything wrong with it.

"I lived as a bisexual for several years and then I realized that you can't do this without hurting someone. So I had to make a choice, as most bisexuals must do—and I chose to become exclusively homosexual when I was about nineteen. I went quite steady with a girl for over a year, at the same time having male contacts. When I found out she was expecting me to marry her, I knew I had to level with her. She couldn't understand at all and really went to pieces. So it's important to make that decision of who you are. I really believe, as do most of my gay friends, that *we are born this way.*"

And according to the small amount of research we now have, no one can say that he is wrong.

At what age does a person usually find out he or she is a homosexual? How do they find out?

Males and females differ considerably as to when they first recognize their homosexuality. For like their heterosexual counterparts, homosexual women generally appear to realize their sexual needs at a later age than do homosexual men, according to Karlen. Males tend to discover their homosexuality in their teens. Lesbians usually make this discovery between the ages of seventeen and twenty-two, although some do discover their homosexuality as late as sixty, and as early as fourteen.[10] Cindy, you recall, had her first homosexual experience at the age of sixteen.

When a homosexual discovers his sexual identity, he may resist *coming out*, due to the terrible fear and guilt associated with being found out. Men and women both have much to lose—families, friends, education, jobs—should they admit they are homosexuals. Females often don't admit their own sexuality until they are older and are in a secure, independent position where their chances of being socially or financially hurt are lessened. They appear more cautious than males.

Emily, for example, told me, "I think I was homosexual since I was very young. I can remember playing *house* with another girl when I was only five or six. I would be the daddy and she the mother. We would undress each other and examine each other's bodies.*

"My mother never worried that I was always with other girls, never with boys. But when I was sixteen, I fell in love with a girl who was twenty-one. We kissed and fondled each other's breasts, but that was all. One day my mother caught us together and from then on I was watched. If I didn't have

---

*Just because a young girl may prefer the companionship of girls, and a boy prefer boys, it does not mean they are homosexual. It is very common for children to prefer being with others of their own gender—and for them to examine each other's bodies and to play *house* and *doctor*. Since most children do get involved in this kind of play in the process of growing up and learning about their bodies, boys and girls should not think they automatically will become homosexual due to this type of childhood behavior. Likewise, adolescent boys and girls are likely to have *crushes* on members of their own sex, and this does not mean they are latent or potential homosexuals.

a date with a boy, I didn't get to go anyplace. So I tried hard
to make it with fellows. At eighteen I got married, but after
a while I couldn't stand having sex with my husband. Now at
twenty, I have met another woman who is thirty and married. We began with a very beautiful friendship. After six
months we both realized we wanted more than friendship.
We are now lovers. My husband is divorcing me. My parents
are completely disgusted with me. But I have to be me."

Men are more likely to discover their homosexuality in
their teens. Their friends begin to date girls, and they begin
to find other interests, or, feeling like outcasts because they
have no interest in girls, they become isolated. Most likely
during their later teens and early twenties they begin to go to
homosexual bars and other places where they can meet
others of their kind. They begin to feel more at ease and less
guilty about their sexual preference and find their way into
the homosexual life-style.

Don, for example, told me, "I think I must have been
nine or ten when I first began to wonder about myself. I
remember my father telling me that I should have been a
girl because I never seemed to like boy's activities, like
playing baseball and football. I liked to help my mother
with her cleaning and cooking. But as I got older, my mother
wouldn't let me do any of these *girlish* things and kept telling
me to go out and play with the boys. I didn't like it, but for
a while, just to please her, I did play baseball. After I left
high school, I started to meet some other gay guys, and from
then on things just started to happen. I really enjoyed being
myself—a homosexual. I was with people who enjoyed the
same things I did. No longer an outcast, I felt cared for and
well liked."

Tim is very typical of male homosexuals. He told me that
he began to have sex with men at age sixteen. "I remember it
was my junior year at high school and I was going with a girl.
I began to think of men, fantasizing about them sexually—
occasionally while with my girlfriend. Even when I kissed
her I thought about how it would be kissing men, and sex

with her became less and less enjoyable. It was then that I
started to go to gay bars with other friends (for fun, as we
called it) and became fascinated with the idea of going to bed
with a man. I began to frequent the bars more and more
often—my only source of finding a lover or a *trick* for the
night.

"Now at nineteen I really have little contact with the gay
scene. Since high school, I haven't been going to bars often,
and my lover and I do other things we enjoy. I'm not one of
these men who always needs to go to social events and parties. Last time my lover and I were at a party was six months
ago. Some of the books you read on sex have always as-
tounded me with the way they picture gays. You read that
we are always looking for new sex partners and a real love
commitment is never there, for we are always *on the make.*
I hate that cliché because I have had one lover for two years.
I loathe the idea of going out to bars and sleeping with different people each week as I did when I first *came out* as a
homosexual. My lover and I have a real commitment and love
for one another and would have it no other way. Of course,
like heterosexual men, some homosexual men do like to *trick*
on a nightly or weekly basis with new partners. That's not
for me."

What kind of sex do homosexuals engage in?

The same as heterosexual—kissing, petting, everything but
sexual intercourse as heterosexuals practice it. We have discussed oral sex in previous chapters. This is the kind of sexual
behavior that many homosexual men and women engage in.
They also may enjoy masturbating each other. Men may also
experience anal sex, that is, a man has sexual intercourse by
inserting his penis into his male partner's anus or *behind.*

When making love, homosexuals engage in kissing and
caressing each other's bodies in the same fashion as do
heterosexuals. However, from the literature one can make
certain observations. Lesbian lovemaking appears to be more
gentle, caring, and committed. Before they experience sex

with each other, they usually develop a feeling of affection. On the other hand, gay male sex is often spontaneous, more intense, immediate, and less committed. Of course, some men, like women, require at least a feeling of friendship before they become interested in sex, and eventually most men enjoy a commitment to another person. But generally speaking, men, straight or gay, are far more able to disassociate sex from love and affection than are women, straight or gay, and can enjoy sex for purely physical release and fun.

Roy tells how it feels to be a homosexual. *"Coming out* was terrific. By the time I was eighteen I was ready, and I had no trouble with the homosexual scene. I was young, attractive, and sexed-up. Sex was easy and enjoyable. At first, it was oral sex and mutual masturbation. But later on I discovered multiple sex with three or four guys, and I loved it."

Amy said she felt somewhat embarrassed talking about her sex life as a lesbian, but she finally agreed. "The love life between two women is very similar to that between a man and a woman. In addition, I think we have much more empathy toward each other. Because we are the same sex, we naturally know what pleases our partner. Women enjoy gentle, loving, touching as their bodies are explored, and we are the more gentle sex. Holding, talking, kissing, caressing have always been important to women. When my partner slowly undresses me and begins to massage my body and to caress my breasts, I just want to go to bed with her. When we have oral sex, I go wild with excitement, and then I enjoy doing the same to her. We aren't interested in each other just for sex. Lesbians usually will have a feeling of affection for each other before they ever get around to having sex."

What does the term coming out mean?

According to homosexuals I have talked with, this concept of coming out has many levels of meaning. It can mean the point at which a person has a sexual experience with a member of the same sex and thus recognizes he enjoys a homosexual relationship. It can mean an *acceptance* of one's homosexuality, either before or after an actual sexual experience with a gay partner. Coming out can also mean the time when a homosexual announces to friends, family, the world, that he or she is gay.

For example, Tom told me, "Coming out to me was when I was able to get up in the morning, look in the mirror and say, 'Hey, you're all right—in fact, I like you!' I feel no overwhelming need to inform my parents of my sexuality. I spent enough time getting over guilt feelings—I don't wish my parents to lay guilt trips on themselves because of the belief that familial relations are the sole cause of one's sexuality. If the time comes when I feel they can share the joy of my own self-acceptance, then maybe it'll be time to tell them. I don't flaunt my sexuality, nor do I try to hide it. I try to accept people for what they are, and expect the same in return."

Where do homosexuals go to make contact with each other?

One of the major problems gay people face is finding a meeting place where they can feel free to mingle. This is not possible in the usual places where the general public gathers.

As Harold said to me, "I can take you to the airport and kiss you goodbye and even shed a tear at your leaving. But when I see my lover off at the airport we must conceal all of our true emotions—to kiss each other farewell would be considered offensive and even obscene by the general public."

The homosexual male or female can behave toward each other according to their real emotions only in privacy or in special places where gay people gather. The usual places are gay bars, discos, baths (usually restricted to males over twenty-one), and a few secluded gay beaches. If a homosexual is not into the "bar scene" his access to potential partners is limited. Homosexual friends have described these meeting places for me.

Baths. Their use by male homosexuals is comparable to the use of massage parlors and houses of prostitution by straights. And in the same way, baths run the gamut from being extremely elegant to very sleazy, and they are found in most large cities. A typical bath will have three floors or levels. On the first level, one may find a health club with athletic facilities such as handball, volleyball, or basketball courts, exercise rooms, and showers. On the second floor, steam baths, saunas, massage parlors, and rooms for group sex might be located. And on the third floor one might find private rooms for intimate sex with a partner. The main difference between a house of prostitution and a bath is that in the latter, a man doesn't pay an individual for sex. He pays for use of the facilities but not for a sex partner, for those in attendance are there to exchange sexual favors. Everyone there desires strictly sexual contact with another, with no intention of developing a friendship or emotional relationship. Multiple partners in one evening is not unusual.

Very few gays go to the baths on any sort of regular basis. Sometimes a gay just happens to be in town alone and decides to try the baths for sexual contact, probably for the same reason a straight married or single man might decide to visit a house of prostitution. Often a gay will go to a bath house following the break-up of an emotional affair as a way to compensate for his hurt feelings or his anger, just as a straight might go to a massage parlor or seek a prostitute for an evening of solace.

Bars. Most gay bars have a homogeneous mixture of "types and preferences." In large cities, bars usually establish a clientele of people with certain preferences—"chicken bars," where younger and older men meet for a sexual relationship; "leather bars," where a person who needs to inflict physical violence on another to become sexually aroused (a sadist), goes to find a person who needs to be physically punished to become sexually aroused (a masochist); "butch bars," where strictly masculine men meet for sexual contact; "lesbian bars" for women; "piano bars," which provide an intimate environment for couples and others not necessarily interested in new sexual contacts; and "discos," which are usually divided into lounge and dance areas.

Those who frequent bars are more likely to want more than a "one-night quickie," as compared with those who frequent baths. Gay bars are often a good source for friendships, as are neighborhood bars for straights.

Gay beaches. Beaches provide an "earthy" setting for contacts. They are usually very difficult to locate, as it is done by word of mouth. But they do provide a setting other than bars for conversation and contact.

Cruising. Cruising is practiced by both straights and gays for virtually the same purpose—looking for a possible date. Window shopping, walking through parks, and grocery shopping are a few "cruise areas."

At sixteen, I have a notion that I am more interested in boys than I am in girls. Am I a homosexual? What should I do? My father would just about die if he ever thought that I was a homosexual. All he ever thinks about is what a great football player I am going to become.

At sixteen, still being more interested in boys than girls and thus doubting one's sexuality does not necessarily mean one is gay. Most youngsters have a natural curiosity about sex and wonder and daydream about what it's like. And it is normal to fantasize about homosexual behavior, especially when one is just being made aware of the whole subject.

Adults, too, are curious about homosexuality. Since little is actually known about how one's sexuality is developed, many myths and untruths have grown into gross generalizations about homosexuals. It is very difficult, knowing the prejudice that exists, not to fear the possibility that you may be a homosexual.

You will not know for sure until you discover that you really have a sexual preference for boys and become sexually involved with them. For now, I think you should make a deliberate attempt to date girls. With practice you may find that you do prefer their company. If you continue to want to be with boys, then you should consult with the Public Health Department or mental health clinic in your community. They will refer you to someone with whom you can discuss your concerns.

Ray makes another suggestion: "If you are, you are. But don't talk about it until you've decided for yourself that you really are interested in boys more than girls. Why upset everyone if you're not sure yourself? Contact the gay crisis line. It's anonymous. Discuss your feelings. Don't let anyone force you into being something you're not, whether that's a football player or a homosexual."

Al expressed a slightly different view: "What you seem to be saying is you want to talk to someone, but not your father, because he may get upset since you are not going to live up to his expectations. Try talking with a clergyman, a doctor, or the public health department in your town. Discuss what you think and feel.

"The feelings we have for others vary. We are attracted to friends, both girls and boys. But the difference is to what extent. A situation may arise in which you could misread your feelings. For example, a close friend may be dating and spending most of his time with his new girlfriend. You feel alone. Jealousy arises! How can a friend be jealous of his buddy's date? It is because he has a strong feeling for his friend. Should he be ashamed to admit it? Guilt probably confronts him. Such a situation can be misinterpreted. Maybe you felt threatened by your male friend's interest in girls and the fact that he is not spending as much time with you as you would like. It is natural for a sixteen-year-old boy still to want only the company of his male buddies. I didn't date a girl until just recently, and I am eighteen. So the entire question needs much discussion and inward examination. Find someone you can trust and discuss your feelings."

Jim rounds out the variety of feelings expressed by the college men: "You should find out for sure which you are interested in. If it is boys, it is not your father's problem. It's your life and you must decide for yourself. Your father may be hurt, but you can't live your life for someone else. And being interested in boys rather than girls should in no way affect your ability as a football player."

Your concern about your parents' feelings if you are a homosexual is well founded. Parents always hope their children will grow up to fall in love, marry, and perhaps give them grandchildren. If this does not happen, they worry about what they have done wrong. In other words, if they find out you are gay, your parents probably will feel they have failed and that you have rejected everything they stand for. Like most homosexuals, chances are that unless you know that your parents can handle the truth, you probably will never let them know that you are gay.

I am heterosexual and I have just found out that a close friend of mine is a homosexual. How should I treat him? Should I tell him to get lost, or what?

Eric expressed a typical feeling of many males I've queried when he said, "I know that I would not treat that person meanly, but I have to say honestly that I would drift away from that friendship. I understand that some people are born with this 'problem' and that that's the way they are. I feel sorry for them 'cause I think it must be harder than hell, living a secret life. I know I couldn't handle knowing this about my friend, so this is why I would drift away."

Joe expressed another view: "If the friendship is deep, I would probably stand by him, but maybe not as closely as before. If he would make any sexual overtures, then it would be time to tell him to get lost. Remember, there is a danger. If my friend's secret became public knowledge, people would look at me and wonder."

Rick had a softer view: "If the friend wants to talk about it to someone, I think you should listen. Explain how you feel—that you are not interested in sharing his way of life. You must accept each other on those terms. Respect how he feels, and he will respect you. But if you found out this information about your friend from someone else, you had better check the source of information before you react."

The college girls I spoke with did not seem threatened by homosexuality. Ruth expressed a typical view: "Treat her the same as always. There is no reason for telling a friend to get lost because she is a homosexual. Would you tell a friend to buzz off if she didn't have the exact same taste as you do in everything else? She just has a different sexual preference; she's not going to change everything else about herself. Why end a friendship if you enjoy a person? But if she started to push her views of homosexuality on you, or propositioned you to have sex with her, then I would discontinue the friendship."

A close friend told me he loved me and said he wished I would consider having sex with him. I was so shocked I just told him to get lost and I haven't spoken to him since. Did I do right?

Many of the students I queried agreed they would have done the same thing. Mike said, "If you are not a homosexual, why associate with him? I probably would have been so mad at such a suggestion, I would have belted him."

Other males expressed Tom's view: "I would definitely say no to that person. I would feel kind of angry at that moment but would not hold this against the person. I probably wouldn't let it bother me later. I would forget about it!"

Jane expressed the typical female response: "What's wrong with a homosexual looking for a possible sex partner just as straight guys do? If they don't ask, they won't find anyone. I think guys are overly sensitive about this. Maybe being asked by a gay guy makes straight men feel like they are girlish, and so they get angry at that, too."

Phil, who was propositioned by a homosexual, had this to say: "I knew this guy casually, and one day when I was looking for my buddy, he invited me into his dorm room at college. He told me I was such a good-looking dude he could really go for me. I was a little flattered until he told me how nice it would be if I would go to bed with him. I was so surprised I couldn't believe my ears. I thought he was putting me on, and I just laughed and told him he must be kidding. He began to explain that sex was pleasant with another man, that I would really enjoy it, and if I wouldn't try, how would I ever know? For some reason, I wasn't angry. I felt as if I were a girl—that is, I was on the other side listening to the same kind of persuasion I use in trying to talk a girl into having sex with me! I kept talking with him, and once he was convinced that I was not the least bit interested in having sex with him he told me to think about it, and he let it go at that. Then we went out and met my buddy, and all three of us had dinner. He acted as though nothing had happened. Well, nothing really had, because he never tried to touch me or force me. If he had done that, I would have punched him out. But I really couldn't get mad at the guy for trying. I do it all the time with girls—sometimes I win, sometimes I lose. Girls don't usually get angry—the ones I really like always say no, and I respect them for that."

It is interesting to note that most of the young men responded in a negative way to the question of receiving a proposition from a male homosexual. As you will see, the women felt better able to cope with a proposition from another female.

I couldn't believe it when one of my very best girlfriends confessed she was a lesbian and asked to go to bed with me and make love. I have been taught that this is very wrong and so I was really scared. I just told her I would not accept it, and now I am having problems with remaining her friend. What would you do in this situation?

The majority of girls who answered this question were sympathetic with the girl who asked the question and were non-condemning of the lesbian. About a third of the girls said they would be upset or scared. Sally expressed the majority view as she said, "I would try very hard not to look too dis-

turbed. I would tell this friend in a nice way that I was not
interested in her offer. I would tell her not to be ashamed for
asking, because this is what she felt she should do. I would
want to have a good heart-to-heart talk in order to gain a
greater insight into each other's sexual feelings. I think the
friendship should be saved if possible. The other girl need
not conform to still stay friends."

Helen added, "I would have to tell the lesbian that I
respect her freedom to have her sexual preference. I would
expect her to respect my sexual preference for males. I would
feel, perhaps, closer to her in a way because she chose to tell
me, but the respect for each other's sexual preference would
have to be upheld if this relationship were to continue. A
person's uniqueness and individuality is of primary importance in any close relationship; any pressure exerted on
the other could destroy the relationship."

In the same light, Janet said, "I would tell her that I
was sympathetic toward her and that I respected her for admitting her homosexuality even though I had never made any
overtures to indicate that I was gay. I think it would be important that the girl be made to realize that she is not weird
or to be feared. Yet, I would be pretty scared—no, *very*
scared."

A slightly different emphasis is noted in Mary's response:
"I would tell her that I was not interested since I am not gay.
My feelings would be difficult to explain. Perhaps I might
wonder if there was something about me that would cause
someone of the same sex to be interested. I don't think the
incident would make me feel good, and although she was my
friend, it might be difficult to maintain our former relationship. I would not let her think that I would change my mind."

Similarly, Nancy said, "I would probably care very much
for this girl and I wouldn't want to hurt her. I would want to
reassure her that I still liked her, but that my affection for
her could never be expressed within the context of a sexual
relationship.

"I doubt that we could continue to be close and do
things together as before," she added, "but I would want her

to know that I would always care about her and wish her
the best. If she could resolve her lesbian feelings and accept
my point of view, perhaps our friendship could continue ac-
tively. I don't know how comfortable either of us could be,
however."

"I would like to think I could just say no and remain
friends with her," said Judy. "But I doubt if I honestly
could. I would be afraid, ashamed, and angry. My first instinct would be to get as far away as possible. If my other
friends—especially boys—found out, it would be devastating.

"If I were a really strong person I would be able to look
her right in the eye and tell her what I think. Then I would
hope we could talk and be open and honest with each other.
But I doubt if I could do that, even though I know that openness and honesty would be the best solution. I would not be
able to remain friends with her, knowing she was a lesbian
and interested in me sexually."

The most negative response from the girls was from
Edith: "If a lesbian approached me sexually, I would be in-
sulted and find it terribly repulsive. Our friendship would
come to an immediate end."

We have been discussing the question of what a nongay
girl would do if she received a proposition for sex from a
lesbian. The answers from nongay girls indicate a feeling of
uneasiness about themselves in such a situation, still unknown to them. Now Ruth and Jane, who have experienced
homosexual relations, tell you how they feel about receiving
or giving a proposition for sex.

Ruth is bisexual and she feels that all people are bisexual.
She adds, "I am aware that I can, if necessary, be stimulated
by either a man or a woman. I was involved with a woman
one time and was afraid, but found it a possibility for me.
I really am not comfortable with this part of me and feel
more secure and healthy in a heterosexual relationship. Sex
is still only sex and there is something in a homosexual affair
that I don't like. There is a *dirty* connotation in all oral sex
for me, and doing it with a female is more *dirty*. Hair and
moisture are a problem. But making love between two girls

doesn't necessarily include oral sex. For me, it included only kissing and mutual masturbation to climax. I would suggest, if you went along with a sexual overture from a girl, that you do it as an experiment. If this friend is someone you care deeply about, you might find it to your liking. If you agreed and didn't enjoy the experience, she would understand, since she no doubt cares deeply about you or she would not have asked you."

Jane, who is a lesbian, gives her views on asking a friend to make love: "Propositioning a friend is very different from propositioning a total stranger. I don't think I would ever ask for sex with someone who had been a friend for a long time. I remember a girlfriend of mine who started discussing sex with me and we both agreed that we would feel uncomfortable and different toward each other if we ever even wanted to have sex. I think it is a mistake for a girl to proposition her best friend unless she really has good reason to suspect that she is a lesbian also. If this is the case, then the *risk* is worthwhile, and being close friends, they can discuss the matter and still remain friends."

Most of the girls have responded in a sympathetic manner toward a lesbian asking a friend to *make love.* It appears throughout this discussion on homosexuality that women *are* less threatened by it than are men.

Why do guys feel so hostile toward homosexuals?

"Perhaps embarrassment," suggests Steve.

"We have learned ingrained hatred from our parents, who have always told us that homosexuality is bad," says Alan.

"They just aren't normal, and we don't like it," offers Dan.

Ben was more detailed and understanding in his reply. "Hostility is a reaction because the existence of a homosexual poses a certain threat to a guy's masculinity. How could anyone suggest a male can be less than just that, when the very symbol of masculinity is the ability to be good in bed with women? Well, it happens, and the very idea seems

to threaten guys who are trying to fill a role that hered-
ity and society have assigned men. It could be because
they are not secure about themselves or because they just
do not tolerate another male who does something that
is not on the program for men. Religious taboos could
also be mentioned, since it is not practical for persons of
the same sex to *waste* their sexuality by not contributing
offspring to society.

"I don't feel a sense of hostility toward homosexuals,
but the thought of myself fooling around with a man for
sexual gratification makes me sick. These people are fulfilling
some need they have, and their need is different from mine
because they have been programed in some particular way—
no one seems to know how. Conditioned as we are in our society, we cannot help feeling repulsed by the idea of sex with
a person of the same gender. But to each his own, and I am
very opposed to the prejudice and discrimination exerted
against homosexuals in our society."

Young women saw more underlying psychological motives for this hostility than did the men.

"Their masculinity is being offended," suggested Lynn.
"They are frightened of it—it is a sign of weakness to them."

"Guys may feel threatened because they are afraid of the
homosexual feelings we have all had at one time or another,"
added Charlotte.

"They think it is an insult to their manhood, and they
feel hostile because part of their identity is lost at the
thought of two men loving one another," concluded Emmy.

I believe Charlotte is the most correct in her assessment
of why men feel so hostile toward homosexuals. Many men I
have talked to seem to fear their own latent homosexual
tendencies. There almost seems to be a feeling that "it is
catching," like a dread disease. Part of this fear is caused by
anxiety about the unknown. Add to this the myths and prejudices surrounding homosexuality, and it is simple to understand why men feel hostile toward homosexuality—this could
happen to them, to their children!

Can I be a homosexual but not engage in homosexual acts?

We need to remind ourselves that homosexuality is not a type of behavior but an expression of *preference* for someone of the same sex. Not all homosexuals engage in homosexual acts. In fact, some homosexuals abstain from any sex acts with others, just as many straight people do. They may get sexual release from self-masturbation, which is a healthy outlet practiced by most men and many women.

We also need to realize that some people who are *not* homosexual seek outlets with others of their own sex. Many persons in prison, for instance, will approach or attack a person of their own sex for sexual gratification and be labeled a homosexual when they are not. Outside of prison, they would prefer the opposite sex.

Aren't homosexuals child molesters?

Most people in prison for child molesting are nonhomosexuals who have a sick desire to molest a young person. We have all heard of examples like the following: the lonely grandfather who masturbates his young grandson; the older sister who fondles her sister's genitals; the baby-sitter who forces or entices a youngster to have sex, exacting promises not to tell. But this behavior is known as *paedophilia*, not *homosexuality*. In the schoolroom, seduction of a young girl by a male teacher is probably more frequent than the seduction of young people by a homosexual teacher.[11]

Incest can also be labeled a form of child molesting, when a father or mother sexually assaults his or her own child, or a brother or sister involves another sibling in a sexual act. The child molester's crime is exploitation of children. Such a person definitely needs psychiatric treatment and, of course, should be kept away from children until he or she is cured.

As Michael Schofield points out in his book, the typical homosexual bears little resemblance to the stereotypes. The

stereotypes have grown out of studies made in prisons, specu-
lations made by psychiatrists about their patients, and long-
standing legal and religious sanctions against homosexual
behavior.[12]

Homosexuality is a condition for which there is no
known resolution. Homosexuals who are really bisexual may
find that living and loving someone of the opposite sex is
more comfortable because of social pressures. But the homosexual who is exclusively homosexual cannot be changed,
according to much of the literature I have read. Those who
accept their condition seldom have serious emotional problems or feelings of hostility toward others who are not
homosexual.

Our society discriminates against homosexuals. It makes
them feel like social outcasts. Because of this, the fear of
discovery for many homosexuals causes great anxiety and
agony. Who wants to be isolated from his friends? Who wants
to have to keep a part of his life a secret from family and
friends, or be subject to ridicule and disapproval? Who wants
to think of himself as being *abnormal* or *perverted*—as so
many people label homosexuals—different from what he has
been taught a man or woman *should* be?

It is important to know that homosexuality is not necessarily related to any form of emotional or mental weakness. Sex preference should never determine the worth
of an individual. Most homosexuals are no different from
heterosexuals with respect to most of the nonsexual elements of their lives. Society must learn to fully respect
and appreciate the uniqueness of each individual homosexual man or woman.[13]

As a parent, would you be happy to know your child was
a homosexual? Probably not, given what we have said about
the pressures society puts on the homosexual. But it is to be
hoped that as a parent, you would be able to give your child
the feeling that he is a person worth supporting and loving
whether he or she is a heterosexual, a bisexual, or a homosexual. Everyone needs acceptance as a human being and
needs to feel worthy of love and respect from others.

conclusion

"ISN'T IT TERRIBLE how many high-school girls are getting pregnant these days?" We hear this question repeated over and over by adults, often angrily, sometimes with condemnation, and seldom is the question asked with any real solution in mind. These adults (your parents) should be seeking ways to give you an adequate sex education in order for you to overcome ignorance regarding human sexuality, and to provide a means for coping with sexual needs in a responsible manner.

Throughout this book I have stressed the need for effective sex education while doing my best to refrain from making moral judgments about sexual behavior. I did not believe it my duty to preach to you about whether any particular kind of sexual behavior is good or bad, or to judge the correctness of the attitudes and behavior of the teenagers who shared with me their questions, attitudes, and experiences.

Try as we have, no one has been able to devise a definitive answer that can account for the development of sexual attitudes and differences in sexual behavior patterns among young people. I am certain, however, from my research and from the literature I have read that the relationship between a child and his parent *is* crucial to the way a child learns about sex.

A child who perceives his relationship to his parents as supportive and close is more likely to behave in ways approved by parents than is a child brought up in a cold family environment. Communication is more effective in a loving family relationship, and a child who feels loved generally feels good about his or her sexuality.

It appears then that the family relationship (that is, the behavior the child sees and experiences at home) is very important in shaping sexual ideals. Unfortunately, there seems to be a real communication barrier between parents and children when it comes to talking about sex, even in families where the relationship is warm and close. Not only do parents often find it difficult to talk with their children, but children in turn feel awkward about asking personal questions of their parents. As Mike said, "Most kids I know, including myself, are afraid to ask these questions when they are young and really need to know."

Janis said her mother couldn't talk about sex because, for her, it has always been very hushed up and she is embarrassed about it. "Sex is a private and personal thing, and Mother feels others might get the wrong idea from what she says about it. She is uptight about sex. Her parents never explained anything to her, so now she can't talk about sex either."

It is clear that not many parents know for sure what their kids think about sex or what their son's and daughter's sexual experience has been. From my own talking with students, I can safely say that less than 10 percent of them have serious conversations with their parents about premarital sex. I am sure many parents do wish they were able to talk to their children.

If you are unable to talk to your parents, you might try saying something like this: "Mom, so many of my friends have such weird ideas about sex and are getting in trouble that I want to know the truth so I can tell my friends who can't go to their parents what we should know. I don't want to get involved with sex at my age, when things can get so messy." I think almost any parent would be willing to sit down with you after a statement like this.

Many schools, too, have avoided their responsibility for providing sex education to young people. As Norma said, "I think sex education is great, but high school is a *little* too late to get this kind of information. I was already messed up by the time I was fifteen, and I don't imagine I'm the only one.

"A high-school sex course should just be a review of what we should learn when we're in grade school and before. When you're older you can look at things differently and see new aspects of a situation, and if you have a good, sound background, any new knowledge will only bring a clearer, broader, and better view.

"I myself had no formal sex education—school or family. I learned everything from the guy up the street when I was nine. Fortunately, he had the right facts. But facts aren't the only important thing. A proper respect for sex, and a realization of its beauty, are as important. I didn't get these other important ingredients. When I was sixteen, my grandmother gave me a sex guide for Catholic teenagers, which was a real farce. And it was too late anyway.

"If I'd had a good sex education in school and from my parents, I don't think I would have treated sex so cheaply as I did in high school. And I'd be a lot happier now, because I wouldn't have ugly memories to live with."

Parents are the chief teachers of sex attitudes. A child relates what he learns at home to what he learns elsewhere. A parent, who is closer to a child than anyone, should teach the facts of sex and the proper attitudes. And the example that parents set will be the most influential. The school should only be an added help to the parent. But for the parents who don't fulfill their part of the bargain, the school will have to provide a complete program.

David was not too devastated by his parents' neglect of his sex education: "My parents completely ignored my sexual education until one day in my eighth-grade year when it was announced that my father and I would attend a father and son sex education lecture series. These came and went, and again the subject was shunned at home. These classes were a good move, but simply a first step. Nevertheless, this was considered more than adequate by my parents. This beginning left me with many questions, but although my father

told me to ask him any questions I had, I felt that he didn't
really want me to delve any deeper into the subject. This feeling became ingrained as I was growing up. I wasn't conscious
of it, but I was silently being taught that all sex was *dirty*. I
say *silently* because this was being accomplished not by acts
of commission, such as actually saying that it was dirty, but
instead by acts of omission. My parents simply did not talk
about sex freely or comfortably. So I learned that it was
not acceptable to speak of sex even in an intimate family
relationship.

"Thus frustrated in my attempt to communicate with my
parents, I did two things. First, I withdrew into myself, feeling that an important aspect of my life was being left out.
I remained this way until I discovered that a lot of kids were
in the same situation that I was in. Well, "misery loves company" and I began to get together with friends and we pieced
things together, little by little. This accomplished the super-
ficial part. We all understood somewhat better the workings
of sex, but learning in this environment left out one essential—the attitudes we should hold about sex.

"I was told by my friends what my parents should have
told me early in my development. I was later to learn that
love is the basic essential. Love must be present not only to
maximize enjoyment, but also to prevent anyone from being
hurt; because if you love someone, you will not hurt him.

"Although I may wish that my parents had been more
open and encouraging with me as a child, it is very challeng-
ing to try to overcome my old attitudes toward sex and life
and to build standards for myself that will stand the test of
time and that I will be proud to pass along to children I
might have."

Dick was fortunate in getting a good sex education in
school. He said: "The type of sex-education program that I
had in high school was very liberal. I attended an all-boy
Catholic high school, and, because of this, there was no need
for embarrassment in discussion.

"Our program started the early part of my freshman year
and ended on my graduation. The program was thorough,

to say the least, because we discussed it daily in theology classes. Information received in the class covered every aspect of sex that I know of, and the terminology used in discussion was very casual and to the point. As of this day I have not seen a school with as thorough a course, but this school is private, so there is little regulation along these lines. The school even had night classes for the students' parents, teaching them sex, and, strangely enough, these night classes were so packed that there were waiting lists for them.

"I feel that all high schools should have this type of program. The program should cover everything from early sexual activity as a child, to dating, intercourse (premarital or otherwise), and end with a marriage course. The courses should consist of a large number of free, open discussions, with a great deal of stress placed on eliminating any inhibitions concerning the discussion of sex. These courses should definitely be coeducational."

Perhaps some of you have had the same experience as this young woman: "The extent of my sex education in school was one talk that was given by a nurse to all the senior girls. The senior boys also had one talk by a phys-ed instructor. I call it a talk because it wasn't any more instructive than that. It primarily covered menstruation, and a few brave girls asked questions concerning dating, going steady, petting, and so forth. However, the questions were answered as indirectly as possible. I don't know who was more embarrassed, the nurse or the girls. I believe that one talk was more detrimental than beneficial. At age eighteen, most girls have some ideas (usually incorrect) that they have learned from their girlfriends or boyfriends, in a sort of *catch-as-catch-can* manner. By having only one talk, great emphasis was placed on the occasion. We were all watched as we entered and left the auditorium; everyone buzzed, giggled, or blushed. If sex education were a gradual, regular part of education, this sort of behavior or attitude would not occur.

"I definitely believe in sex education for students. They are going to find out anyway—why not the right way, through proper instruction from qualified instructors?

They would learn about it as it is—not how they believe it to be. This education would help eliminate the problems created by sexual ignorance: promiscuity, VD, high-school pregnancies, marriages that occur too early. Through proper sex education, we could learn that sex is a healthy, fulfilling, and rewarding experience if it occurs at the proper time in our lives.

"I realize it is difficult for parents to initiate a discussion about sex with their children, and even to answer questions asked by their children. I believe if my school had offered sex education, my parents and I could have discussed it, with the class lectures and books as a starting point. It would have made it easier to do, and in an intelligent, unembarrassing manner. I'm convinced that if this had occurred, my parents and I would have a much closer relationship today, and I would be much more able to confide in my mother."

"I also believe it would be beneficial to have sex education available for parents. I truly admit that if I were a parent, I would not know how to discuss sex with my child, but I certainly would appreciate being able to talk about it with a qualified individual so that, in turn, I would be able to discuss the subject with my child intelligently."

Phyllis, too, had very inadequate sex education: "I never had any sex education in high school except a very short study of the menstrual cycle in biology. This has had bad effects on me. I have *grown up* wondering about sex and being afraid of it.

"Most kids want to know more about the sex act itself, I think, although we are also interested in how the body functions and acts and reacts in general, as well as about the sex organs.

"One big drawback is that girls never really learned about boys. The boys learned about the menstrual cycle, but girls were never told anything about the male sex organ. This led to a great curiosity in me and a sort of repulsion from it. This is bad.

"High-school students should also learn not to be ashamed of the body or of the sex act. They should learn about the advantages and disadvantages of premarital sex so that they can make intelligent decisions."

Peggy gives some good suggestions to counter the type of inadequate sex education she received.

"My total sex education prior to high school was a backyard talk with an older neighbor girl. She was about fourteen and I was eleven. My parents told me absolutely nothing about sex or the use of sex. I am nineteen years old now, and they still have not mentioned sex to me. They must assume that I have gained a knowledge of sex and sexual functions.

"I believe this is the greatest error my parents made in my upbringing and education. Sex education must start early in a child's life, and parental ignorance and embarrassment are no valid excuses for not providing this much-needed information. I didn't know where babies came from or how they were created until that backyard discussion. I think this sudden and blunt learning of sex has caused more doubt, anguish, and uncertainty than any other thing in my young life. I learned other things about sex as I grew older, but I wasn't prepared to accept this new information in the right way.

"In high school, the sex education I received was a total waste. I learned things I had known for years, and the things I really needed to know were left out. Also, the sex education in high school didn't start until my junior and senior years. It must start in the freshman year and progress right through the year. In fact, sex education of some kind must start in elementary or junior high school.

"Much sex education is outdated and unrelated to individual needs. Students' questions about sex are put off or even frowned upon.

"Sex education, in my opinion, must begin *in the home.* When a child starts asking questions regarding birth or kissing, he should be told the truth in a simple and healthy manner by *both* of his parents. This type of unified family sex education should continue until the child is on his own. Family sex education is the basic sex education, and all other forms are secondary."

As another student has said, "Sex education in school should begin in about the fourth or fifth grade and continue in greater detail and with more emphasis in latter years. In high school, special emphasis should be made on teacher-student give and take. Teachers should be able to ask questions and answer those of the students. There must be frank and honest discussions on sex and related topics. Guidance and help in regard to sexual matters should also be provided by the school—teachers should not have to be furtive in their attempts to help children with sex problems. Sex education must progress and grow with the individual. Sex education should become part of everyone's total education."

The teenage years are traditionally a difficult period of life. And, in our day, these normal difficulties are compounded by the kind of society we are forced to face, one in which there is an increasing use of alcohol and other drugs on the youth scene, growing promiscuity and divorce, slackening of commitment between people, sex-saturated media, corruption in politics, and tensions between minority and majority groups. What can society expect of its youth? Rather than making moral judgments about your sexual behavior, society should strive to provide you with the tools to cope with the world adults create for you. Two very basic tools are a close, loving parent-child relationship and adequate sex education to help you deal with the physiological, sociological, and emotional aspects of sexuality. These basic tools are up to you to attain—so put on the presssure to get them.

I urge you to *insist* on the right to a healthy attitude toward sex, free from the hang-ups of previous generations. Demand that programs be developed that teach parents clinical information about sex and how to communicate their beliefs and knowledge to their children. Demand that an effective family-life and sex-education program become part of every grade school and high-school curriculum so that teenagers can learn about love, sex, and marriage in an open, factual manner. Begin making your demands known to your parents, to your teachers, to your school board. In this way, you can better assure that future generations will have the kind of sex education you want and need but have often been denied.

notes

Chapter 3. What about Premarital Sex?   *(pages 24–51)*

1. K. E. Davis, "Sex on Campus: Is There a Revolution?" *Medical Aspects of Human Sexuality*, January 1971, pp. 128-142.

Chapter 5. Preventing Pregnancy   *(pages 62–76)*

1. James Leslie McCary, *Human Sexuality*, 3rd edition (New York: D. Van Nostrand Co., 1978), p. 204.

2. McCary, *Human Sexuality*, p. 217.

3. Ibid.

Chapter 6. Single and Pregnant   *(pages 77-104)*

1. Deborah Yaeger, "Out of Wedlock," *The Wall Street Journal*, Sept. 12, 1977, p. 1.

2. Alice S. Honig, "What We Need to Know to Help the Teenage Parent," *The Family Coordinator* 27 (April 1978), pp. 113-119.

3. John Kantner and Melvin Zelnik, "Sexual and Contraceptive Experiences of Young Unmarried Women in the U.S., 1976 and 1971," *Family Planning Perspective* 9, No. 2 (March-April 1977), p. 56.

4. *The School-Age Parent*, Film Strip Produced by Parents' Magazine Films, Inc., in association with the National Alliance Concerned with School-Age Parents (New York, 1978).

5. Gabriel Stieble and Paul Ma, *Pregnancy in Adolescents: Scope of the Problem* (the National Foundation/March of Dimes, Box 2000, White Plains, N.Y. 10602, 1975).

6. Wallace C. Opel and Anita B. Royston, "Teenage Births: Some Social, Psychological and Physical Sequelae," *American Journal of Public Health*, No. 4 (April 1971), p. 61.

7. F. Ivan Nye, *School Age Parenthood*, Extension Bulletin 667, Co-operative Extension Service (Pullman: Washington State University, April 1976), p. 4.

8. Nye, *School Age Parenthood*, p. 8.

9. Nye, *School Age Parenthood*, p. 5.

10. Nye, *School Age Parenthood*, p. 9.

Chapter 7. Living Together versus Getting Married   *(pages 105-117)*

1. Population Reference Bureau, Inc., "Marrying, Divorcing and Living Together in the U.S. Today," *Population Bulletin* 32, No. 5 (Washington, D.C., 1977), p. 34.

2. Nick Stinnett and Sherry G. Taylor, "Parent-Child Relationships and Perceptions of Experimental Life Styles," *Journal of Genetic Psychology* 129 (1976), pp. 105-112.

Chapter 8. Marriage and the Family   *(pages 118-152)*

1. Nick Stinnett and James Walters, *Relationships in Marriage and Family* (New York: Macmillan, 1977), p. 358.

2. Peter J. Stein, *Single* (Englewood Cliffs, N.J., Prentice-Hall, 1976), pp. 65-66.

3. Population Reference Bureau, Inc., "Marrying, Divorcing and Living Together in the U.S. Today," *Population Bulletin* 32, No. 5 (Washington, D.C., 1977), p. 15.

4. Pop. Ref. Bureau, "Marrying, Divorcing and Living Together in the U.S. Today," pp. 10-12.

5. Pop. Ref. Bureau, "The Value and Cost of Children," *Population Bulletin* 32, No. 1 (Washington, D.C., 1977), p. 24.

Chapter 9. What about Homosexuality?   *(pages 153-182)*

1. Arno Karlen, *Sexuality and Homosexuality* (New York: W. W. Norton, 1972), p. 546.

2. Alan P. Bell and Martin S. Weinberg, *Homosexuality: A Study of Human Diversity among Men and Women* (New York: Simon and Schuster, 1978), pp. 81-84.

3. Bell and Weinberg, *Homosexuality*, pp. 81-84.

4. Bell and Weinberg, *Homosexuality*, p. 84.

5. Bell and Weinberg, *Homosexuality*, p. 230.

6. Karlen, *Sexuality and Homosexuality*, pp. 5-24.

7. Bell and Weinberg, *Homosexuality*, p. 195.

8. Michael Schofield, *Sociological Aspects of Homosexuality* (Boston: Little, Brown, 1965), p. 203.

9. C. A. Tripp, *The Homosexual Matrix* (New York: McGraw-Hill, 1975), pp. 76-77.

10. Karlen, *Sexuality and Homosexuality*, p. 547.

11. Bell and Weinberg, *Homosexuality*, p. 230.

12. Schofield, *Sociological Aspects of Homosexuality*, p. 203.

13. Bell and Weinberg, *Homosexuality*, p. 231.

selected bibliography

Chapter 1. Dating

Bach, G. R., and Deutsch, R. M. *Pairing.* New York: Peter H. Wyden, 1970.

Baker, Luther G. "The Personal and Social Adjustment of the Never-Married Woman." *Journal of Marriage and the Family* 30 (1968): 473–79.

Bartz, W. R., and Rasor, R. A. "Why People Fall in and out of Romantic Love." In *Sexual Behavior*, edited by L. Gross. Flushing, N.Y.: Spectrum Publications, 1974.

Bowman, Henry A. *Marriage for Moderns.* New York: McGraw-Hill, 1974.

Coombs, Robert H. "Reinforcement of Parental Values in the Home as a Factor in Mate Selection." *Marriage and Family Living* 24 (1962): 155–57.

Fromm, Erich. *The Art of Loving.* New York: Harper & Row, 1956.

Greene, B. L. "How Valid is Sex Attraction in Selecting a Mate?" *Medical Aspects of Human Sexuality*, January 1970, p. 23.

Haun, David L., and Stinnett, Nick. "Does Psychological Comfortableness Between Engaged Couples Affect Their Probability of Successful Marriage Adjustment?" *Family Perspective* 9 (1974): 11–18.

Macklin, E. D. "Cohabitation in College: Going Very Steady." *Psychology Today*, November 1974, pp. 53–59.

Rogers, Carl R. *Becoming Partners: Marriages and Its Alternatives.* New York: Delacorte Press, 1972.

Chapter 2. Falling in (and out of) Love

Adams, Margaret. *Single Blessedness.* New York: Basic Books, 1976.

Allon, Natalie, and Fishel, Diane. "The Urban Courting Patterns: Singles' Bars." Paper presented at the Annual Meeting of the American Sociological Association, New York, August 1973.

Bowan, Elisha. *How Can I Show That I Love You?* Milbrae, Calif.: Celestial Arts, 1972.

Fromm, Erich. *The Art of Loving.* New York: Harper & Row, 1956, pp. 40–41.

Goode, W. J. "The Theoretical Importance of Love." *American Sociological Review* 24 (1959): 39–47.

Huston, T. L., ed. *Foundations of Interpersonal Attraction.* New York: Academic Press, 1974.

Murstein, B. I. *Love, Sex, and Marriage Through the Ages.* New York: Springer Publishing Co., 1974.

Ramey, James. *Intimate Friendships.* Englewood Cliffs, N.J.: Prentice-Hall, 1976.

Shibles, Warren, and Zastrow, Charles. "Romantic Love vs. Rational Love." *The Personal Problem Solver.* Englewood Cliff, N.J.: Prentice-Hall, 1977.

Stein, Peter J. *Single.* Englewood Cliffs, N.J.: Prentice-Hall, 1976.

Walters, James; Parker, Karol K; and Stinnett, Nick, "College Students' Perceptions Concerning Marriage." *Family Perspective* 7 (1972): 43–49.

van Den Haag, E. "Love or Marriage?" In *Love, Marriage, Family: A Developmental Approach,* edited by M. E. Lasswell and T. E. Lasswell. Glenview, Ill.: Scott, 1973.

Chapter 3. What about Premarital Sex?

Allen, Mary Wood. *What a Young Woman Ought to Know.* Philadelphia: VIR Publishing Co., 1898.

Bankowsky, William S. *Sex Isn't That Simple: The New Sexuality on Campus.* New York: Seabury Press, 1975.

Burgess, Jane K. "The Influence of Family Relationships on the Sexual Behavior of College Students in Norway and the United States." Ph.D. dissertation, University of Illinois, Champaign-Urbana, 1972.

Cooper, Donald L. "Understanding the Drug Menace." *The Bulletin of the Association of Secondary School Principals* 56 (1972): 53–60.

Davis, K. E., "Sex on Campus: Is There a Revolution?" *Medical Aspects of Human Sexuality,* January 1971, 128–42.

Fink, P. J. "Dealing with Sexual Pressures of the Unmarried." *Medical Aspects of Human Sexuality,* March 1970, pp. 42–53.

Fromm, Erich. *The Art of Loving.* New York: Harper & Row, 1956, pp. 40–41.

Hamilton, Eleanor. *Sex, with Love: A Guide for Young People.* Boston: Beacon Press, 1978.

Kennedy, Eugene C. *The New Sexuality: Myths, Fables, and Hang-ups.* Garden City, N.Y.: Doubleday & Co., 1972.

Levin, R. J. "The Redbook Report on Premarital and Extramarital Sex." *Redbook*, October 1975, pp. 38–44, 190.

Mazur, Ronald Michael. *Commonsense Sex.* Boston: Beacon Press, 1968.

Mendelson, J. H. "Marihuana and Sex." *Medical Aspects of Human Sexuality*, November 1976, pp. 23–24.

Ochsner, A. "Adverse Effect of Smoking on Sexuality." *Medical Aspects of Human Sexuality*, March 1976, p. 15.

Reiss, Ira L. *The Social Context of Premarital Sexual Permissiveness.* New York: Holt, Rinehart and Winston, 1967.

Wake, F. R. "Attitudes of Parents toward the Premarital Sex Behavior of Their Children and Themselves." *Journal of Sex Research* 5 (1969): 170–77.

Chapter 4. Venereal Disease

Brown, Abe A. *Venereal Diseases: The Silent Menace.* New York: Public Affairs Committee, 1974, p. 1.

Johnson, Eric W. *VD.* Philadelphia: J. B. Lippincott, 1973, p. 13.

Lasagna, Louis. *The V.D. Epidemic.* Philadelphia: Temple University Press, 1975, p. 13.

McCary, James. *Human Sexuality.* 3d ed. New York: D. Van Nostrand, 1978.

Najem, G. R. "Incidence of VD Among Adolescents." *Medical Aspects of Human Sexuality*, October 1976, p. 117.

Rosato, D. J., and Kleger, B. "Is Cervical Cancer a Venereally Transmitted Disease?" *Medical Aspects of Human Sexuality*, March 1970, pp. 82–92.

Saltman, Jules. *V.D.—Epidemic Among Teenagers.* New York: Public Affairs Committee, 1974, p. 13.

Stiller, Richard. *The Love Bugs: A Natural History of the V.D.'s.* Nashville, Tenn.: Thomas Nelson, 1974, p. 25.

Taub, W. "Sex and Infection: Venereal Diseases." In *The Sexual Experience*, edited by B. J. Sadock, H. I. Kaplan, and A. M. Freedman. Baltimore: The Williams & Wilkins Co., 1976.

U.S., Department of Health, Education and Welfare. *V.D. and You.* Washington, D.C.: Government Printing Office, May 1973, p. 1.

Chapter 5. Preventing Pregnancy

Alan Guttmacher Institute. *11 Million Teenagers: What Can Be Done About the Epidemic of Adolescent Pregnancies in the United States?* New York: Planned Parenthood Federation of America, 1976.

Ashdorn-Sharp, Patricia. *A Guide to Pregnancy and Parenthood for Women on Their Own.* New York: Random House, 1977.

Associated Press. "Abortion Is Safer Than Birth." *Houston Chronicle*, Mar. 24, 1971.

Blufort, Robert, Jr., and Peters, Robert E. *Unwanted Pregnancy.* New York: Harper & Row, 1973.

Bragonier, J. R. "Influence of Oral Contraception on Sexual Response." *Medical Aspects of Human Sexuality*, October 1976, pp. 130-43.

Calderone, Mary Steichen, ed. *Manual of Family Planning and Contraceptive Practice.* 2d ed. Baltimore: The Williams & Wilkins Co., 1970.

Garrity, Joan [J]. *The Sensuous Woman.* New York: Lyle Stuart, 1969.

Gillette, Paul J. *Vasectomy: The Male Sterilization Operation.* New York: Paperbook Library, 1972.

Hatcher, R. A. "Postcoital Measures to Prevent Pregnancy." *Medical Aspects of Human Sexuality*, September 1976, p. 121.

Himes, N. E. *Medical History of Contraception.* New York: Gamut Press, 1963.

Kasirsky, Gilbert. *Vasectomy, Manhood, and Sex.* New York: Springer Publishing Co., 1972.

Klibanoff, Susan, and Klibanoff, Elton. *Let's Talk About Adoption.* Boston: Little, Brown, 1973.

Lader, Lawrence. *Abortion II: Making the Revolution.* Boston: Beacon Press, 1973.

——, ed. *Foolproof Birth Control: Male and Female Sterilization.* Boston: Beacon Press, 1972.

Lieberman, James, and Peck, Ellen. *Sex and Birth Control: A Guide for the Young.* New York: Schocken Books, 1975.

Lindemann, Constance. *Birth Control and Unmarried Young Women.* New York: Springer Publishing Co., 1974.

Luker, Kristin. *Taking Chances: Abortion and the Decision Not to Contracept.* Berkeley: University of California Press, 1975.

Mace, David R. *Abortion: The Agonizing Decision.* Nashville, Tenn.: Abingdon Press, 1972.

McCary, James Leslie. *Human Sexuality*, 3d ed. New York: D. Van Nostrand, 1978.

Pritchard, J. A., and MacDonald, P.C. *Williams Obstetrics*, 15th ed. New York: Appleton, 1976.

Sarvis, Betty, and Rodman, Hyman. *The Abortion Controversy.* 2d ed. New York: Columbia University Press, 1974.

Wood, H. Curtis, with Rubin, William S. *Sex Without Babies.* New York: Lancer Books, 1971.

Wylie, Evan McLeod. *The New Birth Control.* New York: Grosset & Dunlap, 1972.

Chapter 6. Single and Pregnant

Butler, N. R., and Goldstein, H. "Smoking in Pregnancy and Subsequent Child Development." *British Medical Journal* 4 (1973): 573-75.

Cutright, Phillips. "Illegitimacy: Myths, Causes and Cures." *Family Planning Perspectives* 3, No. 1 (January 1971): 26-48.

DeLissovoy, Vladimir. "Child Care by Adolescent Parents." *Children Today*, July–August 1973.

Honig, Alice S. "What We Need to Know to Help the Teenage Parent." *The Family Coordinator* 27 (April 1978).

Kantner, John, and Zelnik, Melvin. "Sexual and Contraceptive Experiences of Young Unmarried Women in the U.S., 1976 and 1971." *Family Planning Perspectives* 9, No. 2 (March–April 1977): 56.

Myers, Ursula. "When Premaritally Pregnant." *The Personal Problem Solver.* Englewood Cliffs, N.J.: Prentice-Hall, 1977.

Nye, F. Ivan. *School-Age Parenthood.* Extension Bulletin 667, Cooperative Extension Service, Washington State University, Pullman, April 1976.

Pannor, Reuben; Massarik, Fred; and Evans, Byron. *The Unmarried Father.* New York: Springer Publishing Co., 1971.

Pierce, Ruth I. *Single and Pregnant.* Boston: Beacon Press, 1970.

Wagner, N. N., and Solberg, D. A. "Pregnancy and Sexuality." *Medical Aspects of Human Sexuality*, March 1974, pp. 44-71.

Yaeger, Deborah. "Out of Wedlock." *The Wall Street Journal.* Sept. 12, 1977.

Chapter 7. Living Together versus Getting Married

Ald, Roy. *Sex Off Campus.* New York: Grosset & Dunlap, 1969.

Hart, Harold H., ed. *Marriage: For and Against.* New York: Hart Publishing Co., 1972.

Kopecky, Gini. "Unmarried—but Living Together," *Ladies' Home Journal* 89 (July 1972): 64-68.

Lyness, Judith L; Lipitz, Milton E.; and Davis, Keith E. "Living Together: An Alternative to Marriage," *Journal of Marriage and the Family* 34 (1972): 305.

Macklin, Eleanor D. "Heterosexual Cohabitation Among Unmarried College Students," *The Family Coordinator* 21, No. 4 (October 1972): 463-72.

Massey, Carmen, and Warner, Ralph. *Sex, Living Together, and the Law: A Legal Guide for Unmarried Couples (and Groups).* Berkeley, Calif.: Courtyard Books, Nolo Press, 1974.

Mead, Margaret. "Marriage in Two Steps." *Redbook*, July 1966, pp. 48-49, 84-85.

Population Reference Bureau, Inc. "Marrying, Divorcing and Living Together in the U.S. Today." *Population Bulletin* 32, No. 5 (October 1977), Washington, D.C.

Reisinger, Joseph C. "Legal Pitfalls of Living Together." *Single* (August 1973): 58, 104-5.

Rogers, Carl R. *Becoming Partners: Marriage and Its Alternatives.* New York: Delacorte Press, 1972.

Stinnett, Nick, and Birdsong, Craig Wayne. *The Family and Alternate Life Styles.* Chicago: Nelson-Hall, 1977.

Yankelovich, Daniel. *The Changing Values on Campus.* New York: Washington Square Press, 1972.

Chapter 8. Marriage and the Family

Marriage

Arisian, Khoren. *The New Wedding: Creating Your Own Marriage Ceremony.* New York: Vintage Books, 1973.

Bach, George R., and Deutsch, Ronald M. *Pairing.* New York: Avon Books, 1971.

Bach, George R., and Wyden, Peter. *The Intimate Enemy: How to Fight Fair in Love and Marriage.* New York: William Morrow & Co., 1969.

Bailard, T. E.; Biehl, D. L.; and Kaiser, R. W. *Personal Money Management.* Chicago Science Research Associates, 1973.

Bernard, Jessie. *The Future of Marriage.* New York: Bantam Books, 1973.

Berne, Eric. *Games People Play.* New York: Grove Press, 1964.

———. *What Do You Say After You Say Hello?* New York: Grove Press, 1972.

Bird, Joseph, and Bird, Lois. *Marriage is for Grownups: A Mature Approach to Problems in Marriage.* Garden City, N.Y.: Doubleday & Co., Images Books, 1971.

Bowman, Henry A. *Marriage for Moderns.* New York: McGraw-Hill, 1974.

Chapman, A. H. *Marital Brinkmanship.* New York: Putnam, 1974.

———. *Put-Offs and Come-Ons.* New York: Putnam, 1968.

Cotton, Dorothy Whyte. *The Case for the Working Mother.* New York: Tower Publications, 1965.

Crosby, John F. *Illusion and Disillusion: The Self in Love and Marriage.* Belmont, Calif.: Wadsworth, 1973.

Cudlipp, Edythe. *Understanding Women's Liberation.* New York: Coronet Publications, 1971.

Curtis, Jean. *Working Mothers.* New York: Doubleday, 1976.

David, Deborah S., and Brannon, Robert, eds. *The Forty-nine Percent Majority: The Male Sex Role.* Reading, Mass.: Addison-Wesley Publishing Co., 1976.

Farrell, Warren. *The Liberated Man: Beyond Masculinity: Freeing Men and Their Relationships with Women.* New York: Random House, 1974.

Filene, Paul Gabriel. *Him/Her/Self: Sex Roles in Modern America.* New York: Harcourt Brace Jovanovich, 1974.

Firestone, Shulamith. *The Dialectic of Sex: The Case for Feminist Revolution.* New York: William Morrow & Co., 1970.

Fisher, Esther Oshiver. *Help for Today's Troubled Marriages.* New York: Hawthorn Books, 1968.

Folkman, Jerome D., and Clatworthy, Nancy M. K. *Marriage Has Many Faces.* Columbus, Ohio: Charles E. Merrill Publishing Co., 1970.

Fromm, Erich. *The Art of Loving.* New York: Harper & Row, 1956.

Gittelson, Natalie. *The Erotic Life of the American Wife.* New York: Delacorte Press, 1972.

Goldberg, Lucianne, and Sakol, Jeannie. *Purr, Baby, Purr.* New York: Hawthorn Books, 1971.

Golden, Boris A. "Honeymoon Sexual Problems," *Medical Aspects of Human Sexuality* 5, No. 5 (May 1971): 139-52.

Gross, Irma H.; Crandall, Elizabeth W.; and Knoll, Marjorie M. *Management for Modern Families.* New York: Appleton-Century-Crofts, 1973.

Hoffman, L. W., and Nye, F. I. *Working Mothers.* San Francisco: Jossey-Bass, 1974.

Kieran, Dianne; Henton, June; and Marotz, Ramona. *Hers and His: A Problem-Solving Approach to Marriage.* Hinsdale, Ill.: Dryden Press, 1975.

Landis, Paul. *Making the Most of Marriage.* Englewood Cliffs, N.J.: Prentice-Hall, 1975.

Lobsenz, Norman. "Why Some Women Respond Sexually and Others Don't." *McCalls,* October 1972, p. 86.

McCary, James Leslie. *Human Sexuality.* 3d ed. New York: D. Van Nostrand, 1978.

Mace, David R. *Getting Ready for Marriage.* Nashville, Tenn.: Abingdon Press, 1972.

———. *Sexual Difficulties in Marriage.* Philadelphia: Fortress Press, 1972.

Mace, David R., and Mace, Vera. *We Can Have Better Marriages If We Really Want Them.* Nashville, Tenn.: Abingdon Press, 1974.

McGinnis, Tom. *Your First Year of Marriage.* Garden City, N.Y.: Doubleday & Co., 1967.

Masters, William H., and Johnson, Virginia E. *Human Sexual Response*. Boston: Little, Brown, 1966.

Millett, Kate. *Sexual Politics*. Garden City, N.Y.: Doubleday & Co., 1970.

Mornell, Pierre. *The Love Book: What Works in a Lasting Sexual Relationship*. New York: Harper & Row, 1974.

Nichols, Jack. *Men's Liberation: A New Definition of Masculinity*. New York: Penguin Books, 1975.

O'Neill, Neva, and O'Neill, George. *Open Marriage: A New Life Style for Couples*. New York: M. Evans, 1972.

Otto, Herbert. *More Joy in Your Marriage*. New York: Hawthorn Books, 1969, p. 62.

Packard, Vance. *The Hidden Persuaders*. New York: McKay, 1957.

Population Reference Bureau Inc. "Marrying, Divorcing and Living Together in the U.S. Today." *Population Bulletin* 32, No. 5 (October 1977), Washington, D.C.

Porter, Sylvia. *Sylvia Porter's Money Book*. Garden City, N.Y.: Doubleday & Co., 1975.

Reeves, Nancy. *Womankind: Beyond the Stereotypes*. Chicago: Aldine-Atherton, 1971.

Rudd, O. J., and Rudd, Roger. "Husbands and Wives: Talking May Be Sharing." *New Catholic World Magazine*, May/June 1973, pp. 125-29.

Sammons, David. *The Marriage Option*. Boston: Beacon Press, 1977.

Satir, Virginia. *Conjoint Family Therapy*. Palo Alto, Calif.: Science and Behavior Books, 1967.

———. *Peoplemaking*. Palo Alto, Calif.: Science and Behavior Books, 1972.

Schafter, Margaret H., and Gillotti, Susan S. *How to Go to Work When Your Husband Is against It, Your Children Aren't Old Enough, and There's Nothing You Can Do Anyhow*. New York: Simon and Schuster, 1972.

Stassinopoulos, Arianna. *The Female Woman*. New York: Random House, 1973.

Stein, Peter J., *Single*. Englewood Cliffs, N.J.: Prentice-Hall, 1976.

Steinbeck, John. *The Winter of Our Discontent*. New York: The Viking Press, 1961.

Steinmetz, S. K., and Straus, M. A., eds. *Violence in the Family*. New York: Dodd, Mead & Co., 1974.

Stinnett, Nick, and Walters, James. *Relationships in Marriage and Family*. New York: Macmillan, 1977.

Wahlroos, Sven. *Family Communication: A Guide to Emotional Health*. New York: Macmillan, 1974.

Wiemann, John M., and Knapp, Mark L. "Turn-Taking in Conversations." *The Journal of Communication* 25 (1975): 75–92.

Family

Apgar, Virginia, and Beck, Joan. *Is My Baby All Right? A Guide to Birth Defects*. New York: Pocket Books, 1974.

Arnstein, Helen S. *Your Growing Child and Sex*. Indianapolis: The Bobbs-Merrill Co., 1967.

Beckman, Linda J. "Relative Costs and Benefits of Work and Children to Professional and Non-Professional Women." Paper presented at the meeting of the American Psychological Association, New Orleans, August 1974.

Bernard, Jessie. *The Future of Motherhood*. New York: The Dial Press, 1974.

Bradley, R. A. *Husband-Coached Childbirth*. New York: Harper & Row, 1974.

Chess, Stella; Thomas, Alexander; and Birch, Herbert G. *Your Child Is a Person*. New York: The Viking Press, 1965.

Dick-Read, Grantly. *Childbirth Without Fear*. 4th ed., revised and edited by Helen Wessel and Harlan F. Ellis. New York: Harper & Row, 1972.

Dobson, James. *Dare to Discipline*. Wheaton, Ill.: Tyndale House, 1970.

Feldman, Harold. "Changes in Marriage and Parenthood: A Methodological Design." In *Pronatalism*, edited by Ellen Peck and Judith Sendevowitz. New York: Thomas Y. Crowell Co., 1974.

Frank, Lawrence K. *On the Importance of Infancy*. New York: Random House, 1966.

Gruenberg, Sidonie Matsner, ed. *The New Encyclopedia of Child Care and Guidance*. Garden City, N.Y.: Doubleday & Co., 1968.

Guttmacher, Alan. *Pregnancy, Birth and Family Planning*. New York: The Viking Press, 1973.

Hoffman, Lois W., and Hoffman, Martin L. "The Value of Children to Parents." In *Psychological Perspectives on Population*, edited by James T. Fawcett. New York: Basic Books, 1973.

Holstrom, Lynda Lytle. *The Two Career Family*. Cambridge, Mass.: Schenkman, 1973.

Lamaze, Fernand. *Painless Childbirth*. Translated by L. R. Celestin. Chicago: Henry Regnery Co., 1970.

Leboyer, Frederick. *Birth Without Violence*. New York: Alfred A. Knopf, 1975.

LeMasters, E. E. "Parenthood as Crisis." *Marriage and Family Living* 19 (1957): 352-55.

Leshan, Eda J. *The Conspiracy Against Childhood*. New York: Atheneum Publishers, 1967.

Liley, H. M. I., and Day, Beth. *Modern Motherhood*. New York: Random House, 1966.

Lynn, D. B. *The Father: His Role in Child Development*. Monterey, Calif.: Brooks/Cole Publishing Co., 1974.

McBride, Angela Barron. *The Growth and Development of Mothers*. New York: Harper & Row, 1973.

Pohlman, Edward. *Psychology of Birth Planning*. Cambridge, Mass.: Schenkman, 1969.

Scanzoni, John. "Sex Role Change and Influences on Birth Intentions." *Journal of Marriage and the Family* 38 (1976): 43-58.

Veevers, J. E. "Voluntary Childlessness: A Neglected Area of Family Study." *The Family Coordinator* 22 (1973): 197-205.

Whelan, Elizabeth M. *A Baby? . . . Maybe*. New York: The Bobbs-Merrill Co., 1975.

Wright, James D. "Are Working Women Really More Satisfied? Evidence from Several National Surveys." *Journal of Marriage and the Family* 40, No. 2 (May 1978): 301-14.

Chapter 9. What about Homosexuality?

Abbott, Sidney, and Love, Barbara. *Sappho Was a Right-On Woman: A Liberated View of Lesbianism*. New York: Stein and Day, 1972.

Altman, Dennis. *Homosexual Oppression and Liberation*. New York: Outerbridge and Dienstfrey, 1972.

Bailey, Derrick Sherwin. *Homosexuality and the Western Christian Tradition.* London and New York: Longman, Green, 1955.

Bell, Alan P. and Weinberg, Martin S. *Homosexuality: A Study of Diversity among Men and Women.* New York: Simon and Schuster, 1978.

Benson, R. O. *What Every Homosexual Knows.* New York: Ace Books, 1970.

Berger, Raymond Mark. "An Advocate Model for Intervention with Homosexuals." *Social Work,* July 1977, pp. 280–83.

———. "Report on a Community-Based Venereal Disease Clinic for Nonsexual Men." *Journal of Sex Research,* February 1977, pp. 54–62.

Bieber, Irving, et al. *Homosexuality: A Psychoanalytic Study.* New York: Basic Books, 1962.

The Body Politic. Gay Liberation Newspaper. 4 Kensington Avenue, Toronto 2B, Ontario, Canada.

Boggan, E. Carrington, et al. *The Rights of Gay People.* The American Civil Liberties Union Handbook. New York: Avon Books, 1975.

Burgess-Kohn, Jane. "Why Parents Today Worry About Homosexuality," *Parents' Magazine,* January 1977, p. 40.

Clark, Don. *Loving Someone Gay: A Gay Therapists' Guidance for Gays and People Who Care About Them.* Milbrae, Calif.: Celestial Arts, 1977.

Come Out! A Liberation Forum for the Gay Community. 725 Ninth Avenue, New York, N.Y. 10019.

Cory, Donald W., and LeRoy, John P. *The Homosexual and His Society: A View From Within.* New York: Citadel Press, 1963.

Dedek, John. *Contemporary Sexual Morality.* New York: Sheed and Ward, 1971.

Ebert, Alan. *The Homosexuals.* New York: Macmillan, 1977.

Ellis, A. *Homosexuality: Its Causes and Cares.* New York: Lyle Stuart, 1965.

Fisher, Peter. *The Gay Mystique: The Myth and Reality of Male Homosexuality.* New York: Stein and Day, 1972.

Focus. A Journal for Gay Women. 419 Boylston Street, Room 406, Boston, Mass. 02116.

Framick, Jeanine; Nugent, Robert; and Oddo, Thomas. *Homosexual*

Catholics: A Primer for Discussion. Boston: Dignity, National Office, 755 Boylston Street 02116.

Freedman, Mark. *Homosexuality and Psychological Functioning.* Belmont, Calif.: Wadsworth Publishing Co., 1971.

Freud, Sigmund. *Three Contributions to the Theory of Sex. The Basic Writings of Sigmund Freud.* Edited and translated by A. A. Brill. New York: Modern Library, 1938.

The Furies. Lesbian/Feminist newspaper. Box 8843, S.E. Station, Washington, D.C. 20003.

Gay. Four Swords, Inc. P.O. Box 431, Old Chelsea Station, New York, N.Y. 10011.

Gay Sunshine. A newspaper of Gay Liberation. P.O. Box 40397, San Francisco, Calif. 94140.

Hoffman, Martin. *The Gay World.* New York: Basic Books, 1968.

Humphreys, Laud. *Out of the Closets: The Sociology of Homosexual Liberation.* Spectrum Paperback, Englewood Cliffs, N.J.: Prentice-Hall, 1972.

Hyde, H. Montgomery. *The Love That Dared Not Speak Its Name.* Boston: Little, Brown, 1965.

Johnston, Jill. *Lesbian Nation.* New York: Simon and Schuster, 1973.

Jones, Clinton R. *What About Homosexuality?* Nashville, Tenn.: Thomas Nelson, 1972.

Katchadourian, Herant, and Lunde, Donald. *Fundamentals of Human Sexuality.* New York: Holt, Rinehart and Winston, 1972.

Karlen, Arno. *Sexuality and Homosexuality.* New York: W. W. Norton & Co., 1972.

Kinsey, A. C. et al. *Sexual Behavior in the Human Male.* Philadelphia: W. B. Saunders Co., 1948.

Kopay, David, and Young, Perry. *The David Kopay Story.* New York: Arbor House, 1977.

The Ladder. Lesbian/Feminist magazine. P.O. Box 5025, Washington Station, Reno, Nev. 89503.

The Lesbian Tide. 1125½ N. Ogden Drive, Hollywood, Calif. 90046.

McNeill, John. *The Church and the Homosexual.* Kansas City: Sheed Andrews & McMeel, 1976.

Marmoor, Judd, ed. *Sexual Inversion.* New York: Basic Books, 1965.

Masters, W. H., and Johnson, V. E. *Human Sexual Response*. Boston: Little, Brown, 1970.

Miller, Merle. *On Being Different*. New York: Random House, 1972.

National Lesbian Information Service Newsletter. Box 15368, San Francisco, Calif. 94115.

Nichols, John, and Clark, Elijah. *I Have More Fun With You Than Anybody*. New York: St. Martin's Press, 1972.

Oberholtzer, W. Dwight, ed. *Is Gay Good?* Philadelphia: Westminster Press, 1972.

Perry, Troy. *The Lord Is My Shepherd and He Knows I'm Gay*. Los Angeles: Nash Publishing Corp., 1972.

Pittenger, W. Norman. *Making Sexuality Human*. Philadelphia and Boston: Pilgrim Press, 1970.

Schofield, Michael. *Sociological Aspects of Homosexuality*. Boston: Little, Brown, 1965.

Sisters. A Magazine By and For Gay Women. 1005 Market Street, Suite 208, San Francisco, Calif. 94103.

Teal, Donn. *The Gay Militants*. New York: Stein and Day, 1972.

Tobin, Kay, and Wicker, Randy. *The Gay Crusaders*. New York: Paperback Library, 1972.

Tripp, C. A. *The Homosexual Matrix*. New York: McGraw-Hill, 1975.

Vida, Ginny, ed. *Our Right to Love: A Lesbian Resource Book*. Englewood Cliffs, N.J.: Prentice-Hall, 1978.

Weinberg, George. *Society and the Healthy Homosexual*. New York: St. Martin's Press, 1972.

Weltge, Ralph E., ed. *The Same Sex: An Appraisal of Homosexuality*. Philadelphia and Boston: Pilgrim Press, 1969.

West, D. J. *Homosexuality*. New York: Penguin, 1967.

Williams, Colin J., and Weinberg, Martin S. *Homosexuals and the Military*. New York: Harper & Row, 1972.

Conclusion

Calderone, Mary S. "The Sex Information and Education Council of the U.S." *Journal of Marriage and the Family* 27 (1965): 533-34.

——. "Sex Education for Young People—and for Their Parents and

Teachers." In *An Analysis of Human Sexual Response*, edited by Ruth Brecher and Edward Brecher. New York: New American Library, 1974.

———. "Sex Education for Children." *Sexology*, April 1971, p. 71.

Dearth, P. B. "Viable Sex Education in the Schools: Expectations of Students, Parents, and Experts." *Journal of School Health* 44 (1974): 190-93.

Gadpaille, W. J. "Father's Role in Sex Education of His Son." *Sexual Behavior*, April 1971, pp. 3-10.

———. "Sadomasochism." *Medical Aspects of Human Sexuality*. September 1972, pp. 155-56.

Gunderson, M. P. "The Effects of Sex Education on Sex Information, Sexual Attitudes and Behavior." Master's thesis, University of Houston, 1976.

———. "The Interrelationships between Four Sex Variables (Sex Information and Sexual Guilt, Attitudes and Behaviors) and 16 Personality Factors." Ph.D. dissertation proposal, University of Houston, 1977.

Kirkendall, L. A. "Sex Education." In *Human Sexuality in Medical Education and Practice*, edited by C. E. Vincent. Springfield, Ill.: C. C. Thomas, 1968.

Levine, M. I. "Sex Education in the Public Elementary and High School Curriculum." In *Human Sexual Development*, edited by D. L. Taylor. Philadelphia: Davis, 1970.

Lief, H. I. "Sex Education in 106 Medical Schools." *Medical Aspects of Human Sexuality*, September 1974, p. 155.

McCary, J. L., and Flake, M. H. "The Role of Bibliotherapy and Sex Education in Counseling for Sexual Problems." *Professional Psychology* 2 (1971): 353-57.

Mace, D. R. "The Danger of Sex Innocence." *Sexology*, November 1970, pp. 50-52.

Malcolm, A. H. "Sex Goes to College." *Today's Health*, April 1971, pp. 26-29.

Poffenberger, T. "Family Life Education in This Scientific Age." *Marriage and Family Living* 21 (1959): 150-54.

———. "Individual Choice in Adolescent Premarital Sex Behavior." *Marriage and Family Living* 22 (1960): 324-30.

Quality Educational Development, Inc. "Sex Education Programs in the Public Schools of the United States." *Technical Reports of the Commission on Obscenity and Pornography*, Vol. 10. Washington, D.C.: U.S. Government Printing Office, 1970.

Rees, Bill, and Zimmerman, Steve. "The Effects of Formal Sex Education on the Sexual Behavior and Attitudes of College Students." *American College Health Association Journal* 22, No. 5 (June 1974): 370-71.

Spanier, G. B. "Formal and Informal Sex Education as Determinants of Premarital Sex Behavior." *Archives of Sexual Behavior* 5 (1976): 39-67.

Spurr, G. A. "Sex Education and the Handicapped." *Journal of Sex Education Therapy* 2, No. 2 (1976): 23-25.

Wright, M. R., and McCary, J. L. "Postive Effects of Sex Education on Emotional Patterns of Behavior." *Journal of Sex Research* 5 (1969): 162-69.

index

THE AUTHOR

Jane Burgess-Kohn teaches family sociology at the University of Wisconsin. The author of many articles on teenage sexuality, she has been active in furthering sex education courses in schools, counseling young people, and teaching community sex education classes for the parents of teenagers. She is also co-author of *The Widower* with her husband, Willard Kohn (Beacon Press, 1978).